022 066

CW01176614

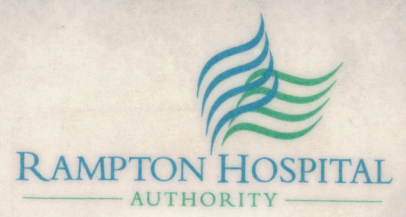

RETFORD
NOTTS. DN22 0PD

TELEPHONE: 01777 24 72 29
FACSIMILE: 01777 24 75 63

SOLD

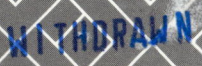

FOR SALE

NORMALISATION IN PRACTICE

NORMALISATION IN PRACTICE

Edited by
Andy Alaszewski and Bie Nio Ong

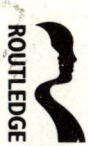

TAVISTOCK/ROUTLEDGE
London and New York

First published 1990
by Routledge
11 New Fetter Lane, London EC4P 4EE

Simultaneously published in the USA and Canada
by Routledge
a division of Routledge, Chapman and Hall, Inc.
29 West 35th Street, New York, NY 10001

© 1990 Crown

Printed and bound in Great Britain by
Billings & Sons Limited, Worcester

All rights reserved. No part of this book may be reprinted or reproduced or utilized in any form or by any electronic, mechanical, or other means, now known or hereafter invented, including photocopying and recording, or in any information storage or retrieval system, without permission in writing from the publishers.

British Library Cataloguing in Publication Data

Normalisation in practice: residential care for
  children with a profound mental handicap.
  1. Great Britain. Mentally handicapped children. care
  I. Alaszewski, Andy II. Ong, Bie Nio
  362.3'088054

Library of Congress Cataloging in Publication Data

Normalisation in practice: residential care for children with a
  profound mental handicap / edited by Andy Alaszewski and Bie Nio Ong.
  p.   cm.
  Includes bibliographical references.
  1. Croxteth Park Project. 2. Mentally handicapped children – Institutional care – England – Case studies. 3. Mental retardation facilities – England – Case studies. I. Alaszewski, Andy. II. Ong, Bie Nio, 1951–   .
  [DNLM: 1. Community Mental Health Services – organization & administration. 2. Mental Disorders – in infancy & childhood. 3. Residential Facilities – organization & administration. WM29.1 N842]
  HV901.G72E546 1990
  362.3'85'083–dc20
  DNLM/DLC   89-24150
                                                                CIP

ISBN 0-415-00598-1

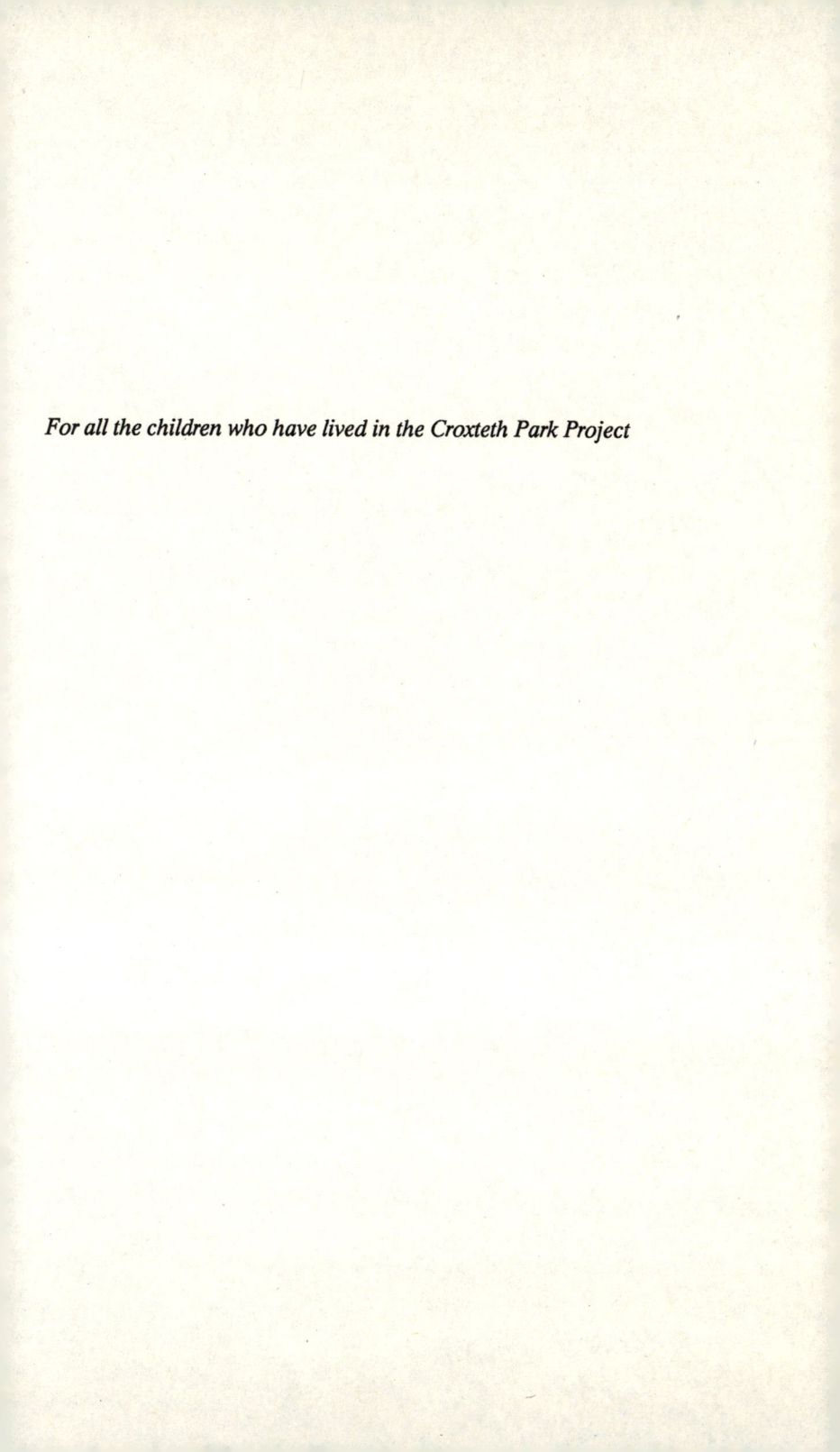

For all the children who have lived in the Croxteth Park Project

CONTENTS

List of Tables and Figures ... ix

List of Contributors ... xi

Acknowledgements ... xiv

Foreword *Gillian Wagner, OBE, Ph.D.* ... xvii

Preface *Andy Alaszewski* ... 1

Introduction *Alan Kendall and Gerry Dodson* ... 7

1. The Development of Residential Care for Children with a Mental Handicap *Andy Alaszewski and Heather Roughton* ... 12

2. Researching the Croxteth Park Project *Andy Alaszewski and Bie Nio Ong with Alan Kendall and Gerry Dodson* ... 30

3. The Selection and Transfer of the Children *Bie Nio Ong and Andy Alaszewski* ... 57

4. The Selection and Training of the Staff *Bie Nio Ong and Andy Alaszewski* ... 76

5. The Selection, Purchase and Conversion of the Bungalows *Bie Nio Ong and Andy Alaszewski* ... 97

Contents

6. Providing Child Care *Andy Alaszewski, Gerry Dodson and Bie Nio Ong* 117

7. Staff Management and Support *Andy Alaszewski, Bie Nio Ong and Heather Roughton* 139

8. Relatives, Neighbours and Volunteers: Mobilising the Informal Sector of Care *Anne Chappell and Andy Alaszewski* 160

9. Education and Health: Co-ordinating Services *Alison Morris and Andy Alaszewski* 182

10. The Psychological Development of the Children *Steven Lovett* 205

11. The Children's Quality of Care *Bie Nio Ong, Nicola Eccles and Andy Alaszewski* 227

12. The Economic Costs *Alan Shiell and Ken Wright* 249

13. Lessons from the Croxteth Park Project *Andy Alaszewski and Sue Hayes* 267

Bibliography 281

Index 296

TABLES AND FIGURES

Table 3.1	Timetable of Main Events Associated with Transfer of the Children from Hospital to the Croxteth Park Project	62
Table 3.2	Shortlist of Children for the First Phase (Nov. 1982)	63
Table 3.3	Selection (Dec. 1983)	64
Table 3.4	Suitability of the Children Admitted According to Senior Personnel	71
Table 3.5	Suitability of the Children Admitted According to Hospital Ward Nursing Staff	73
Table 6.1	Types of Records in the Unit	127
Table 10.1	Classification of Interactive Behaviour in the Objects Scheme Scale	213
Figure 10.1	Sean's Performance on the Bayley Scale	217
Figure 10.2	Sean's Behaviour on the Behavioural Assessment Battery	217
Figure 10.3	Barbara's Performance on the Bayley Scale	219

Tables and Figures

Figure 10.4	Barbara's Behaviour on the Behavioural Assessment Battery	219
Figure 10.5	David's Performance on the Bayley Scale	223
Figure 10.6	David's Behaviour on the Behavioural Assessment Battery	223
Table 11.1	Average Length of Time Taken by Staff to Perform Routine Care Tasks for Each Child (Minutes)	242
Table 11.2	Staff-Child Interactions on a Weekday (Minutes)	242
Table 11.3	Staff-Child Interactions on a Weekend Day (Minutes)	242
Table 11.4	Basic Care Interactions as a Percentage of Total Interactions	243
Table 12.1	The Characteristics of the Two Units and Their Residents	252
Figure 12.1	Hypothetical Comparative Time-Trend of Costs	254
Table 12.2	Use of Medical and Education Facilities	258
Table 12.3	Comparative Average Costs of Continuing Care	262
Table 12.4	Average Costs of Foster Care	264
Table 12.5	Total Expenditure over Three Years	265

CONTRIBUTORS

Andy Alaszewski is Head of the Department of Social Policy and Professional Studies at the University of Hull. He has been involved in research on the development of policies and services for mentally handicapped people since 1972. His doctoral thesis (University of Cambridge) was published by Croom Helm (A. Alaszewski, 1986, *Institutional Care and the Mentally Handicapped*). A revised edition of his survey of services for mothers with mentally handicapped children was published in 1986 (S. Ayer and A. Alaszewski, *Community Care and the Mentally Handicapped*, Croom Helm).

Anne Chappell was a M.Sc. student in the Department of Social Policy and Professional Studies at the University of Hull at the time of her research at Croxteth Park.

Gerry Dodson is currently Assistant Divisional Director in Barnardo's North West Division. He began his social work career in Dunfermline in 1970 and in 1972 moved to Liverpool as a senior social worker. He transferred to Sefton Social Services Department in 1974. In Sefton he developed an interest in staff development and the training field and eventually became the department's Training Officer. In 1983 he accepted the post of Project Leader of the Croxteth Park Project. His interests include supervision, management and mental handicap with a particular emphasis on the ideology of normalisation. He has extensive experience of voluntary work in the field of mental handicap.

Nicola Eccles was a M.Sc. student in the Department of Social

Contributors

Policy and Professional Studies at the University of Hull at the time of her research at Croxteth Park.

Sue Hayes is Assistant Divisional Director with Barnardo's North West Division. She has a degree in social administration and subsequently qualified as a social worker. From 1973 until joining Barnardo's in 1985, she worked for Cheshire Social Services Department, gaining both generic and specialist experience, especially in child care and family work. She has a particular interest in staff development and training matters and is currently undertaking research into aspects of management development.

Alan Kendall joined the North West Division of Barnardo's in 1970 as Assistant Children's Officer (Residential Services). In 1971 he became Divisional Director, the post he now holds. Prior to joining Barnardo's he worked with Lancashire Children's Department as a clerk, Child Care Officer and Assistant Area Children's Officer. He did his social work training at Liverpool University, and holds an M.A. in Social Service Planning from Essex University and a Law Degree from Liverpool Polytechnic.

Steven Lovett graduated in Psychology from the University of Hull. He remained at the University to carry out his Ph.D. in the use of microelectronic learning aids for children with profound mental and multiple handicaps. He has a Masters degree in Clinical Psychology from the University of Liverpool and is presently the Principal Clinical Psychologist for Mental Handicap of Hull Health Authority.

Alison Morris was a M.Sc. student in the Department of Social Policy and Professional Studies at the University of Hull at the time of her research at Croxteth Park.

Bie Nio Ong is the Manager for Research and Development in South Sefton (Merseyside) Health Authority and a Honorary Fellow at the Department of General Practice at the University of Liverpool. From 1983 to 1986 she was a Research Fellow in the Department of Social Policy and Professional Studies at the University of Hull when she worked on the research described in this book. She has spent most of her working life as an academic researching a variety of problems ranging from General Practice to development in the Third World. At the moment she is engaged in putting research into practice by combining research and management in the NHS.

Heather Roughton was a Lecturer in Social Work and the Director of the University of Hull's Programme in Social Work at the time of the Research.

Alan Shiell is a Research Fellow in the Centre for Health Economics at the University of York. His current research interests include economic aspects of the transition to community care and economic evaluation of health service activities.

Ken Wright is a health economist and Deputy Director of the Centre for Health Economics at the University of York. His research programme at York is funded by the Department of Health and is focused on the economic appraisal of policies for the care of people with chronic mental or physical illnesses or disabilities.

ACKNOWLEDGEMENTS

We would like to thank the Department of Health and Social Security not only for their financial support of the Croxteth Park Project and the research project associated with it but also for their continued interest in our work. The initial DHSS support for the research was generous but as and when we needed additional resources for specific aspects of the research, this support was always forthcoming. We enjoyed a close and fruitful relationship with our liaison officers, Sarah Graham and Jenny Griffin, and we would like to thank them especially for their encouragement and support.

We enjoyed working at Croxteth Park and much of our pleasure came from the good relationships we developed with staff in the N.W. Division of Barnardo's, especially Alan Kendall, and Gerry Dodson. As in many relationships, it took time for full trust and confidence to develop, however even in the most tense of situations we were always given the benefit of the doubt. We gained most pleasure out of the final phases of the research when, with Alan and Gerry, we were able to take part in the dissemination workshops. It was a privilege to talk to a variety of audiences about the exciting and successful work that was taking place at Croxteth Park.

Nora Dixon (Barnardo's Co-ordinator of Research and Development) provided essential support for our work. In the early phases of our work she provided us with advice and guidance on the social work issues. She also provided the resources which enabled us to undertake a community study of the Croxteth Park Estate and the facilities for the publication and distribution of the working papers.

During the research many different individuals helped us by

Acknowledgements

providing information. The co-operation we received was remarkable. All the people we approached were willing to see us and provided us with good information, even people whose work practices were challenged by the Croxteth Park Project, for example, the nurses in the long-stay hospitals. We hope that all the individuals who provided us with information will feel that we have made good use of their information in this book.

The children at Croxteth Park figure prominently in our research and in this book. We owe them special thanks for enabling us to learn so much. We were especially impressed in the way in which they persevered and struggled to overcome the many difficulties which they experienced.

We received advice and support from our academic colleagues, especially David Robinson and Gill Manthorpe. Alan Clarke provided invaluable advice on the psychological aspects of our research.

The technical production of this book was a team effort. We could not have done it without the support and tolerance of our colleagues. In particular Petrina Atkinson typed the various working papers on which this book was based and edited the final version. She was always extremely patient and good-humoured. Gill Manthorpe had the tedious task of reading through the book several times. It is thanks to her that we have been able to reduce the typographical errors to a minimum. Our commissioning editor at Routledge, Heather Gibson, was very patient with us.

We started this research in 1983 and in the past six years it has absorbed a significant proportion of our time, sometimes in the evenings and at weekends. Without the support and co-operation of our families it would have been very difficult to undertake this work.

Extracts from the following official publications are reproduced with the permission of the Controller of Her Majesty's Stationery Office:

Curtis Committee (1946) *Report of the Care of Children Committee*, Cmd. 6922, HMSO.
D.H.S.S. (1981) *Residential Facilities for Mentally Handicapped Children, Mental Health Building Pamphlet 1*, D.H.S.S.
D.H.S.S. (1981) *Health Service Residential Accommodation for Severely Mentally Handicapped People: How to Make the Most of Current Design Guidance, Mental Health Building Pamphlet 2*, D.H.S.S.

Acknowledgements

D.H.S.S. (1981) *Care in Action: A Handbook of Policies and Priorities for Health and Personal Social Services in England*, HMSO.

Jay Committee (1979) *Report of the Committee of Enquiry into Mental Handicap Nursing and Care, Vol. I* (Chairman Peggy Jay), Cmnd. 7468-I, HMSO.

Parsloe, P. and Hill, M. (1978) "Supervision and Accountability", O. Stevenson and P. Parsloe, *Social Services Teams: the Practioners' View*, D.H.S.S.

Royal Commission on the Law Relating to Mental Illness and Mental Deficiency (1957) *Report*, Cmnd. 769, HMSO.

Wagner Committee (1988) *Residential Care: A Positive Choice: Report of the Independent Review of Residential Care*, HMSO.

Warnock Committee (1978) *Special Educational Needs: Report of the Committee of Enquiry into the Education of Handicapped Children and Young People* (Chairman, Mrs H.M. Warnock), Cmnd. 7212, HMSO.

Welsh Office (1983) *All Wales Strategy for the Development of Services for People who are Mentally Handicapped*, Welsh Office.

FOREWORD

GILLIAN WAGNER, OBE, Ph.D.

This is an account of a bold and radical experiment to help eleven children with profound mental handicap to leave the sheltered institutional world of hospital life by preparing them at Croxteth Park for placements in families so as to enable them to re-enter the community. It involved not only Barnardo's, D.H.S.S. and the Research Team but relatives, neighbours and volunteers. A measure of the success of the project can be seen in the description of the children as people who have shown "enormous courage, perseverance and determination to overcome their difficulties".

I cannot do better than to quote the final paragraph of the introduction:

> They (the children) have shown that they are capable of taking the love that has been offered them and responding to it. But more than that they have given in equal amounts and have enriched the lives of all who have known them.

In challenging the previously held orthodox view that children with profound mental handicap could only be cared for in a health based facility the Croxteth Park Project has given new hope, not only to the children and young people at Croxteth Park, but, it is to be hoped, to countless others who suffer from the same handicap.

Good ideas quickly perish unless they are researched, documented, published and widely disseminated. There have been other experiments but little research has been published or disseminated in Britain. That is why the publication of this account of the placement of these children, some would say against all the odds, is so important. It demonstrates that the odds need never be all one way again.

It is the vision the Barnardo's staff, the researchers and all who contributed to the making of this book shared, that Croxteth Park should never be assumed to be the final placement for the children, that gives this book its authority, integrity and strength. There is no attempt to minimise the problems and difficulties that were encountered along the way. Each stage of the project is recorded in impressive detail. Through it all shines a belief in the right of every individual to live life to the full.

I am proud to have been invited to write the foreword to this remarkable account of a vision realised through careful planning and perseverance. I hope this book will be widely read and that all who have an interest in the care of people with a mental handicap will benefit from the lessons that have been learnt at Croxteth Park.

PREFACE

ANDY ALASZEWSKI

In this introduction I shall, as director of the research team, briefly outline the structure and objectives of the team.

My first contact with the Croxteth Park Project and the North West Division of Barnardo's came in October 1982 when I received a telephone call from the D.H.S.S. The D.H.S.S. Research Liaison Officer asked me if I was interested in researching a new experimental unit for children with a profound mental handicap. The call came at a time that I was considering my future research plans. I had, since 1972, been involved in researching services for people with a mental handicap. I had supervised a study of the family care of children with a mental handicap and I had undertaken a study of institutional care. I had enjoyed both these studies and both had resulted in major publications (Ayer and Alaszewski, 1986 and Alaszewski, 1986). However I felt rather dissatisfied with our findings. They were mainly negative and critical of the existing pattern of services. For example, the family study showed that mothers were devoted and committed to their children but they received very little support from statutory services. In the light of these relatively negative findings I was considering developing research interests in other areas in which there appeared to be more potential for positive development.

When I received full details of the Croxteth Park proposal, I was convinced that it was an important innovation that could provide a model for other agencies. My research into institutional care indicated that in institutions everyone suffered - patients, their relatives and even the staff. The Croxteth Park Project seemed to offer potential for all the participants to learn and develop. The researchers could play a key part in this process by measuring and assessing the impact of the Project and by examining the processes by which the Project achieved this impact. If we provided a clear account of the Project then other agencies could learn from the Croxteth Park experience and other children, carers and families could also benefit.

As a researcher, I was aware that research imposes costs on the people who are researched. Researchers take information and sometimes provide little in return. I was conscious of the fact that the usual costs of research would be increased by specific characteristics of the Croxteth Park Project - it was a small experimental project with limited funding. Research would be both intrusive and anxiety provoking and could create additional management problems. Therefore the benefits of the research had to exceed these costs.

As an independent researcher I would be able to ask and answer two basic questions about the Croxteth Park Project: "Does it work?" and "How does it work?". The Croxteth Park Project was a bold and radical experiment. The prevailing orthodoxy amongst both health and social work professionals was that children with a profound mental handicap had so many health problems and were so medically fragile that they required long-term care in a health service based facility. The Croxteth Park Project challenged this orthodoxy. It was a community based residential unit staffed by residential social workers designed to prepare children for placement in families.

Senior managers in the N.W. Division were convinced it would work and had persuaded civil servants in the D.H.S.S. that they would successfully care for the children. I also felt that the model looked right and that it should work in practice. However there was a possibility that we might all be wrong and therefore it was prudent to check that the Project did provide the children with good quality care, that the children did benefit in measurable ways from this care and that the cost of providing this care was reasonable.

This type of evaluative research is well developed within disciplines such as psychology and economics. I was fortunate in being able, thanks to special funding by the D.H.S.S., to draw on the skills of a variety of specialist consultants; Steven Lovett (clinical psychologist) monitored the psychological development of the children, Ken Wright and Alan Shiell (health economists) undertook a study of costs of the Project and Nicola Eccles (psychologist) and Bie Nio Ong (medical sociologist) undertook studies of the quality of care. They report on the methods and results of their studies in Chapters 11, 12 and 13.

Since I was relatively confident that the Project would work, I was, perhaps, rather more interested in describing and assessing how the Project worked. When I was researching services for people with a mental handicap in the 1970s, I had identified a major paradox. In some parts of the country practitioners, service planners and families were developing exciting and innovatory schemes.

However these good ideas disseminated slowly. Most people with a mental handicap did not benefit from these innovations. They continued to receive poor quality services organised traditionally. The problem seemed to stem from the fact that the new services were not being adequately researched and documented. Thus agencies, which wanted to modernise their services did not learn from the experiences of innovative services but instead tended to "reinvent the wheel". As researchers, we experienced a similar problem when we started our research. We would have found it helpful to have clear accounts of how other residential projects were set up and operated. This sort of information would have enabled us, as researchers, to identify key issues more quickly, and we could have compared the Barnardo's approach with that of other agencies. Since we started our research the situation has improved with the publication of accounts of the Wessex residential projects (see, for example, Mansell et al., 1987) and the Wells Road Unit in Bristol (see, for example, Ward, 1984a). However, overall the volume of work is still disappointing and it is clear that Mansell et al. experienced problems similar to ours as they cite little British research apart from their own.

Specific evaluative studies such as the psychological study of the children's development can be used to address the "Does it work?" question. However they provide little information on the ways in which the Project achieves its success. To answer the "How does it work?" question, the specific evaluative studies needed to be supplemented with more detailed studies of the processes through which Barnardo's established and operated the Project. These detailed studies were funded by the DHSS and were carried out by Bie Nio Ong with assistance from Anne Chappell and Alison Morris. We describe our overall approach to these studies in Chapter 2 and the results of these studies form the core of this book. In Chapters 3, 4 and 5 we describe and

Preface

assess the processes involved in setting up the Project. In Chapters 6, 7, 8 and 9 we describe and assess the processes involved in caring for the children in the Project. Our description and analysis of the Croxteth Park Project relate to the first three years of the Project, July 1983 to June 1986. Therefore in this book we discuss the children who were living in the Project at the time we collected our data. Many of these children have now moved on to foster care.

As researchers we saw our role as both collecting information and using it. In particular we wanted to document and provide information about the Project, so that other agencies could learn and other children benefit from the Croxteth Park experience. We saw the dissemination as a joint enterprise between the research team and the N.W. Division. As researchers we had skills in collecting, analysing and presenting information, as a voluntary agency, Barnardo's has considerable skills in and facilities for disseminating information. This cooperation forms part of this book. Although the research team has written most of the chapters, staff from the N.W. Division have both contributed to and written parts. In their introduction Alan Kendall and Gerry Dodson set the scene by describing the children and the Project. In Chapter 2 they have contributed a section on their experience of the research. Gerry Dodson contributed to the discussion of the link worker in Chapter 6 and Sue Hayes co-authored the concluding chapter which discusses the lessons which the Division learned from the Project.

This book forms only part of the overall programme of joint dissemination. Other elements include:

* conferences, the researchers and divisional managers have spoken to over 1000 people at conferences and organised study days at:

> *King's Fund Centre*, London, January 1987
> *Cornwall Health Authority*, Truro, February 1987
> *Barnardo's Scottish Division*, Edinburgh, March 1987
> *University of Hull*, Hull, May 1987
> *Barnardo's Welsh Division*, Cardiff, May 1987
> *Cambridgeshire Social Services*, Cambridge, September 1987
> *Barnardo's Irish Division*, Belfast, October 1987
> *Barnardo's Midlands Division*, Birmingham, October, 1987
> *Suffolk Social Services*, Ipswich, January 1988

Cambridgeshire Social Services, Peterborough, June 1988

* pamphlets - over 8,000 distributed

> A. Alaszewski, B.N. Ong and S. Lovett, *Residential Care for Children who are Profoundly Mentally Handicapped*, Dr Barnardo's, 1986.
> S. Hayes and A. Alaszewski, *Setting up a Community Unit: Lessons from the Dr Barnardo's Intensive Support Unit in Liverpool*, Barnardo's 1986.
> G. Dodson and B.N. Ong, *The Link Worker System: An Innovation in Child Care Practice*, Barnardo's, 1987.
> A. Alaszewski and A. Chappell, *The Development of Community Relations on a New Owner-Occupier Housing Estate*, Barnardo's, 1987.
> K.G. Wright and A. Shiell, *Assessing the Economic Costs of a Community Unit: The Case of Dr Barnardo's Intensive Support Unit*, Centre for Health Economics, University of York, Discussion Paper 31, 1987.

* book chapters and journal articles

> R. MacLachlan, "Martin: A Success Story", *Community Care*, 11th December 1986.
> A. Alaszewski and B.N. Ong, "Community Care for Profoundly Mentally Handicapped Children", in N. Malin (ed) *Reassessing Community Care*, Croom Helm, 1987.
> A. Shiell and K. Wright, "The economic costs of a normal life: the case of Dr Barnardo's Intensive Support Unit", *Mental Handicap Research*, 1, pp.91-101, 1988.
> B.N. Ong and A. Alaszewski, "Nurses no longer required", *Nursing Times*, 84, pp. 41-43, 29th June, 1988.

* videos
> *The Art of the Possible*, 1988
> *A Very Special Relationship*, 1988
> *Management: Who Cares?* (provisional title)

If you want further information about the various publications or about the Project contact
Andy Alaszewski
Department of Social Policy and Professional Studies
University of Hull
HULL
HU6 7RX

Preface

Alan Kendall
Barnardo's N.W. Division
7 Lineside Close
LIVERPOOL
L25 2UD

INTRODUCTION

ALAN KENDALL AND GERRY DODSON

The Croxteth Park Project opened in March 1983 when Gerry Dodson, the Project Leader took up his post. But things really got underway when the first group of children arrived in July of that year. With the arrival of the first four children, so began what was to become a most exciting, stimulating and very happy period of our lives. The children are the stars of the show. They have been an inspiration to all of us. Let us introduce them to you:

David was 10 when he moved to Croxteth Park, having spent six and a half years in a hospital. David was to show us what real courage was all about. He was a young man of tremendous determination and good humour. He is one of those people who loves life.

Barbara had spent 7 of her 9 years before she came to Croxteth Park in hospital. She was a normally developing baby up to the age of 13 months. She contracted pneumonia and encephalitis resulting in profound multiple handicaps and severe epilepsy. The first impression she gave us was that of a frightened little girl. She showed little response to those around her. She is now a very pretty young lady whose whole personality shines through when she smiles.

Rob was the youngest person who came to live with us, being four and a half. He had spent all of his young life in hospital. His difficulties were the result of birth trauma. He had the most winning, cheeky smile and sense of fun that openly defied his handicaps. Rob went to live with his new family in 1988.

Connie was 6 when she joined us. She seemed quite unresponsive at first, being content to curl up in the foetal position for most of the day. In August 1984 Connie made history by being the first young person from Croxteth Park to join a new

Introduction

family.

Ivan was admitted to the second phase of the Project in December 1983. He was then an extremely tense 11 year old. He had been in hospital since he was a baby. When approached he would go into spasm but this eased as time passed. He was a young man with large blue eyes and a toothy smile. Ivan brought with him a loving relationship from a lady who had worked with him in hospital. He moved to live with her in October 1985.

Linda was five when she came to Croxteth Park, having spent all of those years in a hospital. We were told she suffered from Cornelia de Lange syndrome. She also had a "lax" oesophagus, and was tube-fed because of this. Linda was a mischievous, delightful little girl who endeared herself to everyone. She moved to live with her new family in 1986.

Mark had spent all of his seven and a half years in a hospital before he came to us. He was a frightened, tense little boy who seemed terrified of people. He had a horrendously severe scoliosis and was permanently in spasm. He was supposedly totally non-responsive. His personality blossomed and he showed courage and determination that was enviable. We were delighted when he joined his new family in September 1986.

Margaret spent 13 years in hospital before coming to Croxteth Park. She had spina bifida, microcephaly and was blind. She was a lovely person who lit-up everyone around her. Her life was dogged by chronic ill-health but despite this she showed enormous courage and her warm personality always shone through. She moved into her new family in December 1984. When Margaret first came to Croxteth Park she was frightened, insecure and unable to accept affection and physical contact, let alone return it. She became confident, and secure in the knowledge that she had a devoted family of her own. She had a close, unique relationship with both parents. Sadly Margaret died in May 1987.

Sean came to live with us in November 1984 aged 11. He had lived in a hospital since he was 7 months old. As well as having severe multiple handicaps, Sean also had periods of severe chest infection. He has large blue eyes that hypnotise you and an infectious laugh.

Stuart moved to Croxteth Park in September 1985. He was 13. He had lived in hospital for 11 years before coming to us. Stuart's birth was normal but subsequently he suffered bronchial pneumonia and encephalitis. His recurrent severe chest infections were life-threatening. He is a slim young man with a crop of curly

Introduction

red hair who loves music of all kinds and enjoys going to concerts.

Anne was almost 16 when she came to us. A tall, slim, attractive young lady who had lived in hospital for many years. A very private person, who loves watching soap operas and listening to music. Anne has standards that are met only in the best restaurants. She is one of those teenagers who enjoys the finer things in life!

Jennifer came to Croxteth Park when she was seven and a half years old. From the age of two she had spells in hospital and when she was three and a half she became a permanent care patient. Most of her early life in hospital was spent apparently sleeping and she was unable to hold her head up unsupported even for a few seconds. She has severe epilepsy but, despite intensive investigation, no specific cause could be found for her mental handicap.

In Croxteth Park, she developed into a happy relaxed young girl who, with help, can enjoy outdoor activities such as camping, visiting the countryside, shopping, swimming and even sledging. She is an exceedingly attractive youngster, who has become an active member of the local Brownie pack where she has established a particular friendship.

These are the most important people in the Project.

Croxteth Park forms part of a range of services provided by the North West Division of Barnardo's for children and young people with a mental handicap, and their families. These activities have been developed by the Division over the last 15 years.

The Division has four projects which support and assist families caring for their son or daughter with a mental handicap at home. Through these projects a variety of support services are offered, including social work support, play schemes, workshops, adventure weekends, respite services, toy libraries, and many others. Through these projects the Division is assisting around 400 families in the North West of England. The Division has six residential projects offering a variety of care - long-stay, short-stay, respite and holiday care. It is into this sector that Croxteth Park fits. Croxteth Park is the latest residential project to be developed.

For over 10 years the Division has been running a fostering service, finding new families for children and young people with a mental handicap. At first most of these children lived within the Division's residential projects. But over recent years children have been placed from other voluntary establishments, local authority

9

Introduction

establishments and direct from hospitals. Children from Croxteth Park have been found new homes and families through the two fostering projects.

The most recent addition to the Division's range of services has been the Advocacy Service. The aim of this project is to provide an advocate for the sons and daughters of parents who we have assisted through the family support projects when their parents are no longer able to do so. This service will also be offered to those young people in foster care who are now adults, and to certain young people in residential care when they too become adults.

In developing these services the Division has been influenced by many people and many other services. High on the list of influential friends have been two agencies in the United States:
* The Eastern Nebraska Community Office of Retardation (ENCOR)
* The Macomb Oakland Regional Centre (MORC) in Mount Clemens, Michigan.

It was MORC that inspired the Division to set up the fostering projects. But it was ENCOR, through its range of residential services, that convinced the Division of the need to provide residential care for children who were profoundly multiply handicapped and medically fragile. Their Developmental Maximation Unit provided a model for such a service. It was on this Unit that Croxteth Park was based.

By the time the Division came to plan the Croxteth Park Project, the principles of normalisation and integration had become part and parcel of the Division's everyday life. In the early 1970s we adopted a fairly pragmatic approach to the ideology based on the belief that normal patterns of everyday life should be available to children with a mental handicap who used our services. This view of normalisation developed from Alan Kendall's experience and knowledge of provision in the United States.

In the early 1980s the principles of normalisation were more formally introduced to the U.K. by a series of normalisation and P.A.S.S. workshops. We responded to these developments by participating in the formation of a small, inter-agency training group in the North West of England which aimed to extend local understanding of normalisation. The work of this training group kept pace with and incorporated contemporary developments in normalisation. In particular the working group was influenced by

Introduction

Wolfensberger's (1983) refinements of the concept. We were particularly influenced by his view that service providers should value people with a mental handicap so that they could compensate for the effect of previous stigmatisation and devaluation. It was particularly important that people with a mental handicap should have their social roles enhanced through, for example, the use of positive imagery.

Our thinking kept pace with these ideological developments and the new residential development at Croxteth Park was to incorporate the principle of normalisation in its practice. The ideology influenced the planning and setting up of the Project, from the choice of houses, the furnishings and decorating of them, the appointment of staff and the training of staff. But most importantly it has influenced the everyday life and running of the Project. Because of our belief in the normalisation principle, and through our growing experience of finding families for our children, we knew that Croxteth Park should never automatically be assumed to be the final, ultimate placement for our children and young people. We knew that no matter how successful the Project was, we could do better for our children, and they would do better, if they were placed with families. Wherever that was possible and desirable, that had always got to be our aim.

We have started with the children. And it is with the children that we must end. They have been an inspiration to us. They have shown enormous courage, perseverance and a determination to overcome their difficulties. They have shown that they are capable of taking the love that has been offered them and responding to it. But more than that they have given in equal amounts and have enriched the lives of all who have known them.

1 THE DEVELOPMENT OF RESIDENTIAL CARE FOR CHILDREN WITH A MENTAL HANDICAP

ANDY ALASZEWSKI AND HEATHER ROUGHTON

In this introductory chapter, we set the scene for our discussion of the Croxteth Park Project by examining the development of theory and practice of the residential care of children with a mental handicap. We divide our account into three sections. In the first we examine the development of residential care within child care services. In the second we consider the impact of these developments on children with a mental handicap. In the third we consider the development of normalisation as an alternative source of ideas for the theory and practice of care.

1.1 THE DEVELOPMENT OF RESIDENTIAL PRACTICE IN CHILDREN'S SERVICES

Before the Second World War the initiative in developing care for children lay with the voluntary agencies, such as Dr Barnardo's and the National Children's Homes, which had, at the end of the 19th century, been concerned mainly with children who had been abandoned by their parents in the growing industrial conurbations. Services were mainly based on residential provision in institutions such as the "village developments" of cottage homes. Barnardo's Barkingside site was a classic example of this form of residential care. Children lived in houses under the care of houseparents. All their social, educational and spiritual needs were catered for in the village community through its homes, school, chapel and community centre. The children's lives were dominated by an institutional regime. For example they often wore a village uniform and were often discouraged from having social contacts outside the community.

The development of child care practice in the post-war period was influenced by the psycho-analytical studies of Burlingham, Freud and Bowlby. Burlingham and Freud researched the institutional nurseries that were set up during the Second World War. They stressed the importance of children's ties to their mothers for their emotional well-being and the damage which resulted from a disruption of these ties (Burlingham and Freud, 1944a and Burlingham and Freud, 1944b). Bowlby in his study of children displaced by the war (1951) argued that the mental well-being of children was dependent on the warm, intimate and continuous relationship with their mothers. He used the term *bonding* to describe the development of this relationship (1965 and 1979). In an article originally published in 1940 he stated that:

> Prolonged breaks in the mother-child relationship during the first three years of life leave a characteristic impression on the child's personality. Such children appear emotionally withdrawn and isolated. They fail to develop loving ties with other children or with adults and consequently have no friendship worth the name. (cited in Bowlby, 1965, p.39)

These studies were extremely influential in the development of child care practice. However, they had two, rather contradictory, effects on the development of residential care. They provided an impetus to and theoretical rationalisation for a change in the pattern of residential provision for children. If residential care was necessary, it should be provided in small community-based, residential facilities which would function as substitute homes in which children could develop warm supportive and stable relations with substitute parents. However, the work of Freud and Bowlby also tended to marginalise the role of residential care. Care outside the family was second best.

In 1944, Lady Allen of Hurtwood initiated a public debate about the nature of child care by publishing a letter in *The Times* calling for a public inquiry. She suggested that many children in care were

> isolated from the main stream of life and education, and few of them know the comfort or security of individual affection. (cited in Heywood, 1978, p. 230)

This debate was given added impetus in 1945 by the death of Dennis O'Neill while in the care of foster parents. The government decided to appoint an inter-departmental committee chaired by Miss Myra Curtis to review the care of children who had been deprived of normal home life.

The Committee broadly endorsed the finding of researchers such as Freud and Bowlby. They found that institutional care had a damaging effect on the development of children. For example, the Committee found:

> in many Homes.... a lack of personal interest in and affection for the children which we found shocking. The child in these Homes was not recognised as an individual with his own rights and possessions, his own life to live and his own contribution to offer. He was merely one of a large crowd, eating, playing and sleeping with the rest, without any place or possession of his own or any quiet room to which he could retreat. Still more important, he was without the feeling that there was anyone to whom he could turn who was vitally interested in his welfare or who cared for him as a person. The effect of this on the smaller children was reflected in their behaviour towards visitors, which took the form of an almost pathological clamouring for attention and petting. In the older children the effect appeared more in slowness, backwardness and lack of response, and in habits of destructiveness and want of concentration. Where individual love and care had been given, the behaviour of the children was quite different. They showed no undue interest in visitors and were easily and happily employed in their own occupations and games. (Curtis Committee, 1946, para. 418)

The Committee felt that care in a substitute family through adoption or "boarding out" was the best option for children who could not be cared for by their parents. However, it accepted that such placements were limited and therefore:

> the need for institutional care must be faced, with the aim of making it as good a substitute for the private home as it can possibly be. (Curtis Committee, 1946, para. 476)

It was important that this care should provide children with the "warmth of affection and motherliness" (para. 344). Therefore the Committee recommended the establishment of small family group homes of a maximum of eight boys or girls.

The main recommendations of the Curtis Committee were implemented in the 1948 Children's Act. The Home Office took over responsibility for the development of services for children who had been deprived of normal home life. Children's Departments were established in local authorities to provide leadership in the provision of child care.

The new Children's Departments generally accepted the case against large institutions and in the 1950s developed alternatives. The group home model was one alternative that was particularly popular in the North-West of England. Heywood, in a history of child care, described these homes in the following way:

> They are mostly to be found on post-war housing estates and they are indistinguishable in appearance from the rest of the houses there. They accommodate eight or less children who are in the care of a married house-mother paid by the local authority and whose husband goes out daily to his employment as a father normally does... These small Homes ... have the advantage of providing care which is very similar to that given in the foster-home - close feeling with the parent substitutes, closer attention to the personal difficulties of the children, and more consistent handling of them than can be provided in the larger Children's Homes. (Heywood, 1978, pp.170-1)

Although some Children's Departments developed group homes as an alternative to large institutions, in others the emphasis was on family placement through adoption or fostering. Initially the preference tended to be pragmatic; family placement was cheaper than residential care. However in the 1960s the criticisms directed at large institutions were increasingly directed at all residential facilities. As Jones pointed out in 1979:

> From the 1950s onwards a new orthodoxy was becoming prevalent to the effect that residential establishments of all kinds were incurably institutionalizing and that we would therefore do better to try to keep people out of them. (cited in Potter, 1986, p. 5)

Prosser summarised attitudes towards residential care in the mid 1970s in the following way:

> in terms of bringing up children in circumstances that approximate most closely to those of a normal family, residential care would seem to offer the most costly and least beneficial alternative. (Prosser, 1976, p.25)

Morris (1984) has traced the development of attitudes and policies in the 1970s from a position in which the family was seen as the *best* locus of care to one in which the family was seen as virtually the *only* locus of care. Morris cited as an example of this shift the following statement by Adcock made in a British Association for Adoption and Fostering publication:

> No child should be deprived of an opportunity to grow up either in his own family or in a new family which he can legally call his own, unless there is a very strong reason to justify this. (Morris, 1984, p.11)

Within social work, residential care tended to be marginalised. The main emphasis was on field work such as preventative work with families and the family placement of children. Residential placement was seen as primarily short-term; either to assess children or to prepare them for family placement. Only children who were difficult to place would require longer-term residential care. This marginalisation can be seen in report of the Seebohm Committee (1968). The Committee placed its major emphasis on the development of services with a community orientation. It "said little about residential work and even less about training for it" (Barr, 1987, p. 38).

By the 1980s, residential workers had lost self-confidence. The Barclay Committee on the role of social workers said it had seen "much evidence of competent, imaginative and innovative practice" (1982, p.55) and cited the pioneering work of Barnardo's in the 1970s. However it also accepted that there were serious problems, including the predominance of fieldwork assumptions, the assumption that family life is necessarily best, the high level of staff turnover and low proportions of staff with formal qualifications.

The Barclay Committee suggested that the dominance of fieldwork assumptions meant the contribution of residential workers to the care of clients was often undervalued:

> When residential services are planned or evaluated the central importance of tending and nurturing ... is often overlooked. Sometimes treatment is regarded as the sole function of an establishment rather than as one component of life for those within it. Reviews of residents' progress may be dominated by fieldwork assumptions and thinking, playing down the insights of residential staff into personal

The Development of Residential Care

issues such as religious choice. (Barclay Committee, 1982, p.56)

The Barclay Committee also challenged the view that family life is always best:

> Despite the emotional damage that may be caused within nuclear families, these family units are generally esteemed more highly than "institutions" by the public and fieldworkers. The saying "a bad home is better than a good institution", simple, yet misleading, still has its adherents. It is possibly for this reason that fostering is assumed unquestioningly to be better than other substitute placements, even though many residents in homes, including some we met, do not share this view. (Barclay Committee, 1982, p.57)

It felt that residential care had a particular role to play, especially for

> a number of deeply damaged children who cannot cope with the demands of fostering, and who can best be helped by very highly skilled residential work over a number of years. (Barclay Committee, 1982, pp. 69-70)

Despite the recommendations of the Barclay Committee, residential work remains marginalised in most social service departments. The Social Services Select Committee in its 1984 report on children in care saw the position in the following way:

> Residential care is going through an intensely difficult period, which may be optimistically typed as being a process of transition but less optimistically viewed sometimes looks like a gradual process of destruction. (cited in Potter, 1986, p.4)

In 1985, the Secretary of State responded to the widespread anxieties about residential care by asking the National Institute for Social Work to set up a committee of inquiry. The Committee provided the following description of state residential work:

> The Review was set up at a time when there was wide agreement that residential services, particularly in the statutory sector, were in a demoralised state, too often used as a service of last resort and seen to be of low status. (Wagner, 1988, p.1)

The Development of Residential Care

Comment

The development of child services has gone through distinctive phases. In the 19th century concerns about the care and control of children led to the development of institutional care. These institutions came to be seen as a problem and the next phase was the development of alternatives. Initially the alternative was smaller residential facilities but more recently it has been seen as community services such as family placement. In the next section we shall show that services for children with a mental handicap have gone through similar phases, albeit at a slower place.

1.2 THE DEVELOPMENT OF CARE OF CHILDREN WITH A MENTAL HANDICAP

Until 1971 the services for children with a mental handicap had different financial, administrative and legal frameworks from services for other children. While Children's Departments of local authorities were moving away from the institutional provision of residential care in the late 1940s and 1950s, mental handicap hospitals remained the basis of residential provision for children with a mental handicap. Indeed as late as 1975, Tizard estimated that

> in England and Wales about one-fifth (9,200 out of an estimated 45,000) of all severely subnormal children are in institutional care; 7,400 in mental subnormality hospitals and 1,800 in local authority, voluntary or privately run hostels. (Tizard, 1975, p.53)

Successive governments were aware of the damaging effects of institutional care on children with a mental handicap. For example, the Curtis Committee found the existing provision for children with a mental handicap was "one of the most serious problems we found in our visits" (Curtis Committee, 1946, para. 509). Similarly the Chief Medical Officer of the Ministry of Health in his annual report for 1956 commented adversely on the effects on children of institutional care and stated that these children needed

> love, security, companionship and stimulation if the love,

> security, companionship and stimulation if the personality is to develop normally. (cited in Shearer, 1980, p. 53)

However, during the 1950s the accepted view was that the needs of children with a mental handicap were so distinctive that they were better met through special services such as mental handicap hospitals. For example, although the Royal Commission on the Law relating to Mental Illness and Mental Deficiency urged that attitudes to children with a mental handicap "should certainly be more like those in other child care and education services" (1957, para. 329), it accepted the maintenance of segregated services.

In the 1960s researchers, particularly Tizard, challenged the accepted view that children with a mental handicap benefitted from segregated services. For example, Tizard monitored the effects on children with a mental handicap of a move from a traditional mental handicap hospital to a small community-based unit modelled on a residential nursery, the Brooklands Unit. The results of the experiment were very favourable. The children made marked and significant progress when compared to children who remained in the mental handicap hospital (Tizard, 1964, pp.133-4).

In the late 1960s Tizard reinforced his critique of hospital care in the child welfare project which he conducted with King and Raynes. Tizard argued that the hospital care was inferior to that provided in children's homes. Through a comparative study of different residential facilities, Tizard and his colleagues wanted to show that these unfavourable conditions were not the product of the children's handicaps but were rather the result of the organisational structure of the hospitals. Their central hypotheses were that

> the organisational structure of a residential unit in large part determines staff roles and role performances... (and that) staff behaviour influences the manner in which children behave, and the competencies which they acquire. (Tizard, 1975, p.52)

Tizard and his colleagues found important differences between child care in hospitals and children's homes. The hospitals had complex organisational structures based on long hierarchies. The head of individual units, e.g. ward sisters or charge nurses, had little contact with the children who were generally "serviced" as a group. Children's homes tended to have simpler structures with less hierarchy. The head of the unit was usually involved in child care. The researchers found that these homes offered a warm and supportive environment in which the children were treated as individuals. The homes had many of the features of ordinary family life, i.e. staff and children often ate meals together (King, Raynes and Tizard, 1971).

Tizard and his colleagues clearly felt that children with a mental handicap benefitted from residential facilities modelled on the homes that had developed in mainstream child-care. They felt that the organisational features and staff behaviour in the children's homes accounted for the higher levels of skills they found amongst children in these homes:

> We thought it likely that the greater frequency of conversation to the children by staff, more of whom were available at peak times when the children were in the units, and the fact that the staff ate with the children thus providing an adult model for them to copy, accounted for the higher levels of skill on the part of the children in the child oriented units. (Tizard, 1975, p.64)

The scandals within mental handicap hospitals at the end of the 1960s meant that Tizard's work was sympathetically received in government. Central government encouraged local authorities to develop facilities for children with a mental handicap within the mainstream of children's services and attempted to "humanise" the care provided within mental handicap hospitals. For example, in 1974, the DHSS organised a national seminar to consider ways of improving the quality of life of children and adults in mental handicap hospitals. As a result of this conference it issued a Circular designed to ensure that the hospitals were aware of and met the social, emotional and intellectual needs of the children in their care. The Circular drew heavily on the model of care provided in children's homes, e.g. staff were not to wear uniforms, the units were to have daily routines that were as close as possible to those of a normal home and the children were to have space for their own clothing and possessions.

Thus in the early 1970s there was an emphasis on integration. Services for children with a mental handicap were to "catch up" with those for other children, where possible through the use of the same services and where not through the development of services modelled on those provided for other children. This emphasis on integration can clearly be seen in the reports of the Court and Jay Committees. The Court Committee (1976) was established to review the provision of health services for children. The Committee felt that long-term care for children with a mental handicap was inappropriate as all children should share the same services. The Committee stated that children with a severe mental handicap

> have more in common with other children because of their childhood than they do with severely mentally handicapped adults because of their common disability. (Court Committee, 1976)

The Jay Committee (1979) on Mental Handicap Nursing and Care accepted the views of the Court Committee. It stated that all children with a mental handicap should have the right to experience normal life and that no child should have to live in a long-stay hospital. If children could no longer live with families then they should live in small, locally based residential facilities which provided normal life experiences.

Although many aspects of the Jay Committee report received a lukewarm response from Ministers, they did accept the Committee's view that children with a mental handicap should not live in mental handicap hospitals. In 1980 the Secretary of State for Social Services stated:

> The time has come to state unequivocally that large hospitals do not provide a favourable environment for a mentally handicapped child to grow up in ... I can think of no more important aim than to try to ensure that all children who do not need specialised health care have the chance to grow up and develop to the best of their potential in their own homes or in small homes in the community. (cited in Shearer, 1981)

However, the model of care being advocated for children with a mental handicap, was now being questioned for other children. Within children's services, residential services had become a professional back-water. The newly developing residential services for children with a mental handicap could no longer draw on models developed in child care services. They required their own specific model. We shall in the next section discuss one source of this alternative model - normalisation.

1.3 NORMALISATION AND THE DEVELOPMENT OF RESIDENTIAL SERVICES FOR PEOPLE WITH A MENTAL HANDICAP

Normalisation as a philosophy of care for people with a mental handicap developed in Scandinavia at the end of the 1950s as a reaction to the shortcomings of institutional care for people with a mental handicap. Grunewald credited Bank-Mikkelsen with its original formulation and he argued that the rapid spread of the philosophy in Scandinavia in the 1960s was associated with its simplicity.

> Normalisation ... could be understood by all personnel, all administrators, and policy-makers. It meant providing the intellectually handicapped with an everyday life and a social environment bearing the closest possible resemblance to normal conditions. (Grunewald, 1986, p.2)

The early advocates of normalisation felt that life in institutions was grossly abnormal, and were concerned to identify alternatives that would provide people with a mental handicap with a normal pattern of everyday life.

In the late 1960s the concept of normalisation spread to the United States, where it was particularly associated with the work of the Eastern Nebraska Community Office of Retardation (ENCOR) and Wolfensberger. In the United States the normalisation philosophy acquired a different emphasis. From being a relatively simple pragmatic alternative to institutional care it acquired a rather complex theoretical base and some supporters of normalisation tended to see it almost as a moral crusade.

The moral character which normalisation acquired can be best seen in the concern with the civil rights of people with a mental handicap. Advocates of normalisation argued that institutional care deprived people with a mental handicap of their rights as citizens, therefore it was important to restore these rights through appropriate legislation and services. Stark, McGee and Menolascino, who were associated with the work of ENCOR, argued that their services were based on

> The recognition of the inherent worth and dignity of the mentally retarded person as equal to that of any other person...; yet, because of the nature of their very special needs, there is the concurrent recognition of society's responsibility to provide the types of programs and services needed to support and maintain the person in family and social life. The United Nation's affirmation of the rights of mentally retarded persons is reflected in a myriad of evolving laws in every nation - laws that reaffirm the rights of retarded persons as the same as all other persons. (1984, p.3)

The theoretical elaboration of normalisation was associated with the work of Wolfensberger. He drew on sociological thinking and used sociological concepts to analyse the problems of existing services and to develop an alternative model. In particular he was influenced by sociologists' thinking about the causes of deviance.

In the 1950s and 1960s, sociologists began to challenge the traditional view of deviance and its causes. Traditionally, behaviour of deviants, such as people with a mental handicap was seen as a product of their innate characteristics or handicap. Sociologists argued that it was difficult to distinguish the behaviour of deviants from that of other people before they had been officially labelled or classified. They argued that it was society's reaction that created deviance and the type of behaviour associated with it. Individuals labelled as deviant would, for a variety of reasons, conform to the stereotype of a deviant and would experience loss of status, social value and social stigma. Dexter argued that people with a mental handicap suffered especially from a society's reaction:

> There is... the experience which may be observed over and over again of the denial of employment, of legal rights, of a fair hearing, of an opportunity, to the stupid because they are stupid (e.g. have a low I.Q. or show poor academic performance), and not because the stupidity is relevant to the task, or claim or situation. (Dexter, 1964, p.40)

For Wolfensberger normalisation was a method of reducing deviance by reversing the social processes that create deviance. A mere assertion that people with a mental handicap should live normal lives was not enough. Wolfensberger (1983) argued that as institutions created a set of devalued and stigmatised roles, it was possible to reverse the process and enhance the social roles of people or groups who were at risk of devaluation. He suggested this could be done through the enhancement of the social image and perceived competences of such people. Thus for Wolfensberger it was important that people with a mental handicap be associated with positive images and were given opportunities to be involved in activities that stress their skills rather than their disabilities. This might not initially change handicapped people's skills and abilities, but it would change the way they were perceived and treated and should eventually result in improvements in their skills.

In the 1970s the concepts of normalisation were publicised in England by the Campaign for People with a Mental Handicap (CMH) (See Tyne, 1987). In the early 1970s, the more pragmatic approach tended to dominate. It could be clearly seen in Kendall and Moss's pamphlet published by CMH in 1972. Kendall and Moss argued that segregation created second-rate services:

> A cause and consequence (of segregated services) has been the stigma attached to the mentally handicapped and the separate institutions for them. (Kendall and Moss, 1972,p.7)

They advocated a pragmatic approach to the development of integrated services.

> For the handicapped child, integration offers the opportunity to gain self-confidence and social skills to deal with the outside world and non-handicapped people ... Integration should offer a more normal environment and more relevant and wider social experiences ... It should also enable the mentally handicapped to feel part of, and be part of their local neighbourhood. (Kendall and Moss, 1972, p.8)

This relatively pragmatic approach could also be seen in the work of the influential King's Fund Working Party on an Ordinary Life. The Working Party's emphasis was on providing people with a mental handicap with normal life experiences. It argued that the role of welfare agencies was to provide the conditions in which people with a mental handicap could experience such normal living:

> mentally handicapped people have the same rights and, as far as possible, the same responsibilities as all other members of the community. They also have the right to the additional help they may need to claim the common rights of

> the citizen... Those who serve mentally handicapped people have a duty to ensure that opportunities to live life to the full are available to them. (Towell, 1980, p.14)

The more theoretical approach could also be identified in England. For example, Race in his account of normalisation drew heavily on Wolfensberger's later work. He argued that normalisation was concerned with the social processes that create deviance and in particular:

> the imposition of social roles by people on one another, and the resultant reinforcement of stereotyped behaviour in that role... Normalisation is not seeking to blame people for using language which ascribes social roles, or for providing services in environments and in ways which produce these roles but ...(seeking) to break into the circle of role ascription: (a) by realising it is there; (b) by altering the circumstances which perpetuate it. (Race, 1987, pp. 66-67)

Race identified some of the ways in which more positive roles could be developed and used. People with a mental handicap were at high risk of acquiring negative social labels. Therefore it was important to minimise this risk by:

* providing them with the best physical appearance;
* providing them with greater opportunities for valued behaviour;
* generally veering to the "conservative" side of appearance and behaviour (adapted from Race, 1987, p.70).

Race stressed the importance of "valued social participation". Race argued that it was not the activity but where and how that activity took place and was perceived that was important. For example, swimming in a hospital pool involved participating in a segregated and devalued activity. Taking part in a "special" swimming lesson with a class of children from a special school might result in physical integration but did not involve the valued social participation that resulted from swimming at the same time as other members of the public.

The Jay Committee was influenced by the pragmatic approach to normalisation and developed a model of care based on this approach. The Committee started with a clear ideological statement that specified the individual rights of people with a mental handicap. For example, the Committee stated that "mentally handicapped people have a right to enjoy normal patterns of life within the community" (para. 89a). The Committee argued that services should be fitted to people not people to services:

> We preferred to consider each individual as having a unique constellation of general and special needs which were unlikely to be met by trying to match a particular group of residents to a particular kind of building. (para. 99)

The Jay Committee was critical of all purpose-built residential facilities and felt that there was a tendency for all purpose-built facilities to be institutional:

> We are beginning to realise the influence of architecture on the nature of the social environment and we need to investigate whether the style of the new purpose built homes for mentally handicapped people is in fact perpetuating the old "institutional" approach to care. (para. 114)

Similarly the Committee argued that

> A purpose built unit on the outskirts of a housing development or a town is not in our view "in the community". (para. 135)

To ensure that mentally handicapped people had a right to enjoy normal patterns of life in the community, the Jay Committee recommended that all residential facilities for mentally handicapped people should be provided in "ordinary houses, suitably adapted for those with additional physical handicaps" (para. 135). The preference of the Committee was "for such homes to be in specially adapted private houses" (para. 114). Although the Committee accepted the need for more specialised regional or sub-regional accommodation, it felt that

> wherever possible these homes should share as many of the characteristics of normal living which we envisage in our staffed local homes as possible. (para. 147)

In their description of the role of residential staff they emphasised the importance of individualised care:

> The staff must be able and encouraged to see each child as someone for whom their whole thrust of care is directed

towards the development of all their capabilities to the fullest potential. (para. 118)

The Committee felt there was a link between unit size and the care which residents received:

> whereas a 40 bed ward was regarded as small by comparison with a 70 bed ward 15 years ago, many people now think of "small" as meaning a maximum of 6 children in a house ... In this home (as envisaged by the committee) the small group of familiar people who care for him will provide opportunities for the child to develop emotionally ... socially and intellectually. (paras. 114 and 117)

In its discussion of the organisation of the residential facilities, the Committee stressed the importance of the normal experiences of everyday life. The Committee felt that "mentally handicapped people should be able to develop a daily routine like other people" (para. 91h). The Committee saw the provision of normal life experiences as a central feature of the new residential units.

> The small unit which we envisage is a place where residents and staff live together as a unit, a place where meals are cooked, washing-up is done and tradesmen are seen. In such small homes ... the child will experience as normal a life as possible ... the contribution of those in the surrounding neighbourhood will be of high importance, and neighbours, shop-keepers and friends will play their part. We want the children to see the milkman and, however small they are, to be taken out shopping. This means that the social unit is one in which the staff are not enclosed but share many aspects of daily living with the children. (paras. 116 and 119)

Comment

Normalisation is compatible with models of social work practice and residential care. For example both are based on views that children should have normal life experiences and should be treated as valued individuals. However normalisation can be seen as a broader and more aggressive model of care. It is broader because it is not restricted to children. It is more aggressive because it starts from the moral proposition that people with a handicap have a right to a normal life and services should be

The Development of Residential Care

judged in terms of the ways in which they provide opportunities for such a life. Although normalisation is most closely associated with the development of services for people with a mental handicap, there is some evidence that it is beginning to influence services for other groups. For example, it is possible to recognise aspects of the normalisation philosophy in the report of the Wagner Committee discussion of Principle of Practice in residential care (1988, pp.60-69), in particular in its emphasis on the right of people in residential care and in its emphasis on the importance of normal life experiences for people in residential care.

1.4 SUMMARY AND COMMENT

The development of current thinking about the residential care of children with a mental handicap has been influenced by developments within child care in general. Prior to the Second World War the dominant pattern of care for all children who could not be cared for in their families was the institution, e.g. the village development. In the 1940s researchers and policy-makers accepted that this form of care damaged children's emotional development because it deprived them of mothering. In the 1950s the initial response to this research and thinking was the development of group homes which provided children with "substitute" parents and a "substitute" family. In the 1960s these homes themselves came under criticism and the emphasis shifted to preventative work with family and foster care. Residential care became a back-water in child care and social services.

Initially the separate legal, administrative and financial framework of services for children and mental handicap services meant that there was little cross-fertilisation of ideas and practices. This was particularly evident in the 1950s. At the time Children's Departments were dismantling large institutions, the health service was investing in mental handicap hospitals.

The cross-fertilisation started in the 1960s and was particularly associated with the work of Tizard. In the Brooklands experiment at the beginning of the 1960s, he showed that the models of child care that had developed with their emphasis on developing close relationships between the staff and the children could be used to care for children with a mental handicap and were a better form of care. He reinforced the results of the Brooklands study with the Child Development Studies which he undertook at the end of the 1960s with King and Raynes.

In the early 1970s the evident failure of institutional care for people with a mental handicap resulted in a major change in policies. The emphasis shifted from segregation and the separate development of services to integration. Policy-makers were keen to integrate services for children with a mental handicap with services for other children, where possible, and where it was not, to model services for children with a mental handicap on services provided for other children. Thus they drew heavily on models of child care developed within residential settings.

However, these models were being criticized and in some cased abandoned within child care. This created a vacuum. In the late 1970s this vacuum was filled by the development of the normalisation philosophy. This philosophy provided a framework within which new forms of residential care could be developed.

2 RESEARCHING THE CROXTETH PARK PROJECT

ANDY ALASZEWSKI AND BIE NIO ONG
WITH ALAN KENDALL AND GERRY DODSON

As the Croxteth Park Project was innovatory, it was appropriate that it should be researched using an innovatory style of evaluative research, the ethnographic approach. In the first section of this chapter the researchers (Andy Alaszewski and Bie Nio Ong) set the ethnographic method in context by discussing styles of research. In the second section the researchers discuss evaluative research of services for mentally handicapped people. In the third section the researchers discuss the relationships involved in our research. In the fourth section, Alan Kendall and Gerry Dodson provide their account of the research process.

2.1 STYLES OF RESEARCH

Social research can be defined as the collection, analysis and use of information about people and society. Everybody is a researcher and without research people cannot exist. Most human action is research based and involves the individual in processing information. However, everyday or low-level research can be differentiated from more specialist and high-level research.

Everyday researchers collect information because they have a particular purpose. If the information is wrong, inadequate or inappropriate then the everyday researcher relatively quickly suffers the consequences. In contrast, specialist researchers should not have a personal stake in the information collected, they do not need it to accomplish some practical activity. The purpose for which the data is collected is often not self-evident. Everyday research is usually short-term and the researcher can form judgements about the utility and accuracy of the information he or she is collecting and using. In contrast, specialist research is usually long-term and there is usually a long time lag between the identification of the purposes of the research, the collection of the data for the research and the use of the information. It may be difficult to assess whether the information collected is appropriate for the purposes of the research. There are often no built-in safeguards or cross-checks in specialist research as the researcher does not usually directly experience the consequences of wrong, inadequate or inappropriate data.

Many of the activities and decisions that the everyday researcher can take for granted need to be made explicit by the specialist researcher. For example, whereas the everyday researcher does not have to be explicit about the purposes of his or her research, the methods of data collection and the use of information, the specialist researcher should be explicit about these aspects of the research. The specialist researcher therefore adopts a distinctive role as a researcher.

Different styles of research can be differentiated by the different ways in which the researchers define their role. In experimental research, researchers define their role in the same way as natural scientists. They see the people they are researching as the "objects of the research". These researchers tend to use the preferred natural science approach to data collection - observation. Their main methodological preoccupations are to find methods of measuring the human behaviour which they observe and devising experiments to test hypotheses about this behaviour. This style of research is best developed in psychology laboratory experiments (see for example, Milgram, 1974).

Most social scientists accept that the people involved in research cannot and should not be treated in the same way as chemicals in an experiment. Instead the social researcher needs to recognise that his or her subject matter is unique and needs to be investigated in special ways (See for example, Barnes, 1976, p.2). Researchers who recognise the uniqueness of human subjects, differ in the way they define their research role.

Social survey researchers tend to see research as a one-way process in which the researcher defines the basis of the research relationship and collects information from the subjects of the research. In the social survey, information is collected from a sample of a population using a standard set of questions in either a questionnaire or an interview. The researcher aims to minimise interviewer bias (see for example, Sellitz et al., 1965, pp. 583-4).

Researchers using an ethnographic approach argue that the social factors should not be treated as extraneous "noise" or bias which the researcher seeks to minimise. They should be accepted as part of the research process. The researcher should develop a more complex relationship with the people he or she researches and should not accept the limited and artificial relationship which is necessary for the "one-off" interview. The researcher should seek to participate more widely in the social life of the people who are being researched and should try to understand the basis of their social actions. This approach is best developed in ethnographic fieldwork (Sieber, 1982, p.1). Central to the success of the ethnographic approach is the relationship which the fieldworker establishes with the people he or she is studying. Only when a relationship of trust exists will the researcher start to find out how the members of a culture experience their world and begin to understand the meaning of the various actions he or she observes.

Thus the central problem in ethnographic research is how to establish and maintain a relationship of confidence and trust between the researcher and his or her informants. In a social survey the basis of the relationship is informed consent but informed consent means that the researcher defines the nature of the research. Wax argues that ethnographic research should be based on equality and parity between researcher and researched and on reciprocity (Wax, 1982, p.46).

Researchers undertaking experimental or survey research use specific research instruments. The reader of a research report has a clear account of how the data was collected and whether this type of data will provide an appropriate answer to the research question. Researchers using the ethnographic approach do not use a single or limited set of research instruments. Therefore it is difficult for the reader of an ethnographic report to assess whether the researcher has succeeded in establishing a relationship of trust and whether he or she has really understood his or her informants.

There are two ways in which the ethnographic researcher can give the reader confidence in the research. The ethnographic researcher can write reports based on detailed data so that the reader can judge and assess the quality of some of the raw data. The ethnographic researcher can give the reader the feel of the data by subjecting it to minimal alteration, e.g. by giving long extracts from interviews.

The ethnographic researcher can also present a natural history of the research and explain how he or she developed a relationship with his or her informants. This natural history is a biographical and intellectual account of the development of the research and was pioneered by Whyte (Whyte, 1955). After we have discussed the specific problems of adapting the ethnographic approach to evaluative research we shall provide a natural history of our research.

2.2 EVALUATING SERVICES FOR MENTALLY HANDICAPPED PEOPLE

In Britain the dominant approach to the evaluation of services for mentally handicapped people has been either experimental or based on social surveys of care organisations.

Tizard's study of the Brooklands Unit (1964) was a landmark in evaluative studies. His research approach was modelled on the experimental technique. Tizard was convinced that mental handicap hospitals did not provide an environment which stimulated the development of young children with a mental handicap and that small units based in the community and run along the lines of residential nurseries would. To prove this he established a small residential unit, Brooklands, and transferred a group of children from a traditional mental handicap hospital into the unit. He then assessed the impact of these two contrasted environments by comparing the emotional and psychological development of the children in Brooklands with that of a control group of children who stayed in the hospital. His impressionistic account of the success of Brooklands (pp.133-4) was substantiated by psychological observations of the children's development, in particular the linguistic development of children with Down's Syndrome (Lyle, 1960).

In this experiment, the researchers established roles as neutral observers who had to exclude extraneous factors or bias. For example, they needed to ensure that the group of children transferred to the new unit were properly matched to the control group that stayed in hospital so that the changes in development and behaviour could be attributed to the change in the environment, and not to any intrinsic differences in the children. Similarly they needed to establish procedures that would record and measure the changes that did take place. Thus the main concerns of the researchers were in selecting and matching the children and in developing ways of measuring the change. There was little discussion of the relationship of the researchers to the other participants.

Although Smith and Cantley (1985, pp. 6-8) argue that evaluative studies of health and welfare services have been dominated by the experimental approach, in the field of mental handicap the survey approach has also been important (Morris, 1969, King, Raynes and Tizard, 1971 and Raynes, Pratt and Roses, 1979). Tizard, Sinclair and Clarke (1975) have argued that the survey approach is not only the best approach to evaluative studies it is also the only approach that yields meaningful results. They argued that only in survey studies can the researcher really exclude extraneous social factors.

Perhaps the most sophisticated survey of services for people with a mental handicap was Raynes, Pratt and Roses's study of the care provided in three large institutions in the United States (1979). Raynes, Pratt and Roses were scrupulously careful in the development of their research instruments. They were particularly concerned about methods of measuring the quality of care provided in the institutions and the different variables which might affect the type of care provided. These included resident characteristics and difference in organisational structure.

As in most survey studies there was relative silence on the social context of the research. In their preface, Raynes, Pratt and Roses briefly described the funding of the project and acknowledged the assistance of the various agencies and staff but this was not discussed in any detail. They acknowledged that the institutions were "an integral part of a complex set of relationships involving competing participants with varying degrees of power and influence" (p.20), but they never outlined the position of the researchers within these relationships.

Some aspects of such diverse organisations as mental handicap hospitals, local authority hostels and community units for people with a mental handicap can be compared. For example, it is possible to compare the different costs per resident, the quality of care which residents receive and the psychological development of residents in different types of care setting and, as part of our research, we did undertake such research. But, by itself, this type of comparison may be inadequate, misleading and limited: inadequate because it fails to explain the factors that give rise to the differences; misleading because there is usually an implicit assumption that the organisations being compared have the same objectives and functions; and limited because only specific features of the services can be compared.

Many organisations, even when they provide services for similar clients, provide a very different package of services. The Croxteth Park Project took children from local mental handicap hospitals and therefore it was possible to make some comparisons between the care of the children in the hospitals and the care of the children in the Project. But the differences between the hospitals and the Project were so great that it is doubtful whether the comparisons could totally capture and contrast the differences between the two care settings. In hospital, the children formed a small group of profoundly mentally handicapped children amongst a much larger group of more able and older mentally handicapped people. Any attempt to "explain" their situation in the hospital would have to locate them in the various networks and classifications of the hospital care (Alaszewski, 1986). In the Project the children still had a profound mental handicap but as there were no other residents they did not form part of a system of classification but were the focus of individual care plans. There was a whole range of similar contrasts that rendered comparison difficult.

Although the ethnographic approach to research is well established and yields useful insights into the operation of care organisations such as mental handicap hospitals, it appears to be difficult to use this approach for evaluative research. As the experimental and survey approaches are both comparative, they can be easily adapted for evaluative research. The ethnographic approach seems less suitable. In the ethnographic approach the researcher aims to get inside a culture so that he or she can really understand it. This type of commitment and the need to develop a close relationship with the people being researched are difficult to reconcile with the independence needed for evaluative research. The researcher using the ethnographic approach to evaluation, needs to establish a balance between understanding and judging.

Smith and Cantley (1985) have provided one model for achieving this balance in their study of an innovative psychogeriatric day hospital. In the first part of their research, they tried to understand the various ways in which participants assessed the performance of the day hospital. They identified six separate ways in which participants defined and evaluated the success of the unit. In the second part, they used these categories as a basis for an evaluation of the performance of the day hospital. The bulk of the data was collected, analysed and reported in these six categories. However the researchers did not fall into the trap of imposing a specific meaning on terms such as "free patient flow", rather they used their data to explore the ways in which different participants defined these terms and assessed the organisation's performance in relationship to them.

The approach outlined by Smith and Cantley is one model for ethnographic evaluative research and there are some aspects which we drew on. These included the importance of trying to understand the different objectives pursued by participants, the need to undertake detailed research and the need to present detailed evidence so that ideas and/or actions were assessed in context. However we also had reservations about their approach. They were almost totally reliant on statements made by the various participants. Although this provided a useful way of assessing ideas, it did not help to explore the relationship between the ideas that were expressed in the various statements and the various actions and activities. Rich qualitative interview material can be balanced with quantitative material.

Although we shared Smith and Cantley's general approach and views, we adopted a more structured approach. We were concerned to understand and to identify objectives but we did this for specific aspects of the establishment and operation of the Project. From our reading of the literature, from our experience of other care organisations and from our discussions with our funders in the D.H.S.S. and senior personnel in Barnardo's, we felt that certain key processes would be important in the establishment and operation of the Project, e.g. the selection and training of the staff and the selection and transfer of the children. Each of these processes formed a distinctive topic or theme for our research.

For each topic area we adopted the same approach. Our first concern was to identify the participants' objectives. As this was an evaluative project we gave precedence to the stated objectives of senior personnel, especially as they appeared in various documents. In an innovative project with special support from an outside funder, these stated objectives had a special status and relevance. However, we were aware that these written objectives had to be operationalised and that different participants would have different views about them. We therefore interviewed various participants to assess their view of the ways in which the Project should operate to achieve its objectives. The second stage of our research was a description of the processes by which the Project achieved its objectives. We used a variety of data including records of meetings, observation of meetings and interviews with key participants to document these processes. The third phase of our research in each topic area involved an assessment of the extent to which the Project achieved its objectives. The major part of this assessment was based on statements made by participants about their perceptions of the performance of the Project in each area. However in each topic area we wanted to supplement this with other forms of data.

Comment

Ethnographic research probably makes high demands on the researcher and other participants in the research. The researcher has to self-consciously define a role and then has to explicitly manage the relationship with the people he or she is researching. In evaluative ethnographic research, the researcher is simultaneously trying to understand the views and activities of people and at the same time trying to evaluate and assess them. This can create considerable strain and tension in the relationship.

2.3 DEVELOPING AND MANAGING RELATIONS

Barnes has identified four separate and distinctive groups that have a role to play in social research and refers to them as "citizens", "scientists", "sponsors" and "gatekeepers". Citizens, or in our terminology informants, provide information and their statements and activities form the raw material of the research (Barnes, 1979). The scientists are the researchers who collect, analyse and publish the information. The sponsors provide the resources for the research. These people may be the researchers themselves or a group of citizens but more frequently they are a research council, government agency or private company. The scientists may also need to negotiate with gatekeepers, people who control access to the information that they need (Barnes, 1979, p.14-15).

Sponsors The research was sponsored by the D.H.S.S. The

D.H.S.S. wanted to know if its money was well invested, if it was worth renewing the investment, and in particular, if the Project provided a satisfactory standard of care for children with such profound handicaps. However the D.H.S.S. had more specific interests in the Project. The Project was an alternative model of care. The D.H.S.S. wanted to know whether this model of care could work and if so, what were the implications. The D.H.S.S. therefore was concerned that the evaluation should demonstrate the extent to which the Project's objectives were achieved and the problems associated with their achievement.

Gatekeepers The Project was located in the N.W. Division of Barnardo's and the senior personnel in the Division acted as the gatekeepers. Managers in voluntary agencies are in a difficult position. They do not have secure funding for their activities but depend on the skills of the agency's professional fund raisers and various grants. The Agency had a commitment to research and to the use of research findings. The Agency accepted that research would identify some areas of practice that could be improved. Indeed, if it did not then it would not be particularly useful to the Agency. However researchers are not accountable to the Agency and cannot be controlled in the same way as employees. The Division had a special interest in the success of the Project. Senior divisional managers saw the Project as a logical development of their earlier service innovations for children with a mental handicap and their families. Senior divisional managers, and in particular the Divisional Director, wanted to demonstrate that the principles of normalisation developed in Sweden and the U.S. could be used in Britain.

Informants There were many informants in our research but, as our main sources of information were the children, the staff and divisional managers, we shall concentrate on their interests.

All the children in the Project had a profound mental handicap and in many cases they also had severe physical handicaps. They could not speak and could not articulate and protect their own interests. It was difficult to identify the wishes of these children as they were so handicapped. For children with a profound mental handicap, the concept of informed consent has little meaning or relevance. Although the parents of the children were their legal guardians and could give consent on behalf of their children, in practice the research was part of the overall package and the parents either had to accept or reject the package as a whole. The concept of reciprocity was more meaningful and formed the basis of our relationship with the children. It was asymmetrical reciprocity. The children were a major source of information. In exchange we performed a range of services for the children. We made the children a major focus of our research (for a similar approach see Jones's study of Beech Tree House (1983) a residential school for handicapped children with severe behaviour problems). Our research could also help to protect the interests of the children. To do this it was important to supplement the data produced by the main ethnographic project with data produced by the regular psychological assessment of the children so that we could monitor and assess the children's progress.

The Residential Social Workers (R.S.W.s) and especially the link workers were major informants. The link workers had a complex relationship with the research. On the one hand they saw themselves as protecting the interests of their child and on the other their own actions were part of the research. It is possible to question the extent to which the link workers did indeed protect and further their children's interests.

The link workers were helped and supported by the Project Leader and the assistant project leaders. The Project Leader was responsible for the overall management of the Project and acted as a link between the Project and its environment. For example, he interpreted agency policy for the Project staff and passed on the views of Project staff to senior management. He was the only qualified social worker in the Project and, as such, was the "guardian" of professional social work values in the Project and a major model of social work practice. The Project Leader was particularly exposed in the research process.

Researchers Our backgrounds were very different from those of the other participants. The Research Director had researched services for mentally handicapped people and had an interest in ethnographic research. The Research Worker had experience of research in health settings, developing countries, an interest in feminist and marxist theory and ethnographic research. We did not have a special interest in or commitment to normalisation.

As researchers we were not only interested in practice, we were interested in theory. We were interested in the ways in which the operation of the Project could illustrate general social processes. Thus as we researched the Project we were also engaged in the intellectual process of theorising, i.e. generalising and abstracting. We therefore had to decide what relationship should exist between theory and practice. We decided that theory should provide the tools for the ethnographic research and in so far as ethnographic research helped to refine these tools, this was a useful by-product (Geertz: 1973, p.27). As academics and researchers, we had a commitment to a successfully completed research contract, which could be defined in terms of maintaining a satisfactory relationship with informants, gatekeepers and funders and producing publications that enhanced our reputations and career prospects.

Setting up the Project: Funders and Gatekeepers

In their application for funds to the D.H.S.S., Barnardo's stated that they wanted an evaluation of the Project. The D.H.S.S. accepted Barnardo's proposals and decided to fund such an independent evaluation. In October 1982 the liaison officer from the D.H.S.S. contacted the Research Director to see if he would be interested in undertaking this research. They wanted

> some research which would both describe in detail how the project works and evaluate how far the scheme was able to meet its objectives for the development of the children concerned.

Drawing on the past experiences of research and the requirements of the D.H.S.S., the Research Director prepared a proposal. He decided to use the ethnographic approach to describe the establishment and operation of the Project, assess the extent to which the Project achieved its objectives and disseminate information about the Project. He also stressed the importance of feeding back information to Project staff and managers as quickly as possible so that they could learn from the research and that in turn they could influence the design of the research. He felt this reciprocity was an essential part of the project and argued that the research should have an action research element, i.e. the research should contribute to the operation of the Project and influence decisions made in the Project.

In October 1982 the Research Director sent a proposal to the D.H.S.S. and to the Barnardo's working group. In November he met the Barnardo's working group in Liverpool. It was clear that some of the group did not like the proposed ethnographic research and they were concerned about the objectivity of the research. They were particularly worried about the action research component, which they felt could contaminate the research and could create a bias in the research findings. Their concerns were shared by the D.H.S.S. and the D.H.S.S. did not accept the initial proposal. They sent the Research Director new guidelines that made it clear that there should be no action research.

The Research Director then prepared a revised project proposal that excluded all reference to action research. This proposal envisaged research on three main aspects of the Project: its establishment, its operation and the progress of the children. The research on the establishment and operation of the Project was based on the ethnographic approach, whereas the evaluation of the children was to be comparative using psychological data. In the proposals, the Research Director stressed the importance of the production of and discussion of research reports.

The Department accepted the revised application in March 1983. As soon as the Department and Barnardo's had approved the research proposal and agreed the funding of the project, the second phase of the establishment of research could start, the recruitment of the research worker. Given the scope and range of skills required, the selection of the right researcher was crucial for the success of the project. The D.H.S.S. agreed that a senior person should be recruited and agreed that the appointment should not be restricted to any particular discipline.

The Research Director placed advertisements in the academic press and, from the applications, prepared a short-list of five people. Four of these applicants had a sociology or anthropology background and one a psychology background. To select the best and most acceptable researcher, the Research Director set up an interviewing panel composed of himself, the Head of his Department (a medical sociologist), the Professor of Psychology, a representative from the D.H.S.S. (the liaison officer) and a representative from Barnardo's (an educational psychologist). The panel interviewed the short-listed applicants in June 1983. They agreed that none of the applicants had the necessary combination of skills to carry out the whole project but that two applicants had the expertise and experience to undertake the ethnographic aspects of the research.

Since the interviewing panel could not decide which of the two applicants was best, they decided to consult the staff of the

Project. The interviewing panel agreed that each applicant should be invited to attend a separate study day on the R.S.W. training programme. Both applicants agreed to take part in a training day. At the end of each day, the Project Leader discussed each candidate with the R.S.W.s. They had a clear preference for one of the applicants. She was offered and accepted the post of research worker.

Collecting the Data: Developing a Relationship with Informants

The main objective of the ethnographic part of our research was to understand the working of the Project. To do this we needed detailed information about the Project and we needed to establish close working relations with the Project staff. There were a variety of reasons why this might be difficult. The D.H.S.S. had agreed to fund the Project for three years and then had the option of renewing that funding for a further three years. It was inevitable that the researchers would appear as powerful and even threatening outsiders.

We had, at an early stage, to address the issue of power and how to develop a more symmetrical and reciprocal relationship with care staff. Feminist researchers and researchers in developing countries have addressed the issue of the relative power and status of researchers and researched. They have questioned the myths of ethnographic research in which the researcher is somehow seen as "going native" (Oakley, 1981, Graham, 1983, Nichter, 1984 and Freire, 1985). Real empathy cannot exist as the basis of the relationship is not shared culture. The research worker participates in the culture as a researcher. The research worker dealt with this contradiction by undertaking some activities that established a common identity between herself and the people she was researching and some activities that clearly differentiated her and set her apart as a researcher.

The researcher started to develop her relationship with staff in the Project in August 1983. To establish her identity and share in the experience of setting up the Project, she attended most of the training sessions for the second group of R.S.W.s and regularly visited the Project. She visited the Project on the same basis as members of the Project staff. She spent part of each visit with the staff and children in the living areas. She talked to the staff and answered their questions. Much of this initial talk focussed on the nature of the research. The researcher explained the nature, objectives and process of the research so that she shared her "experiences of being a researcher" (Stanley and Wise, 1983, pp. 166-7). There was anxiety amongst the staff about the research. The researcher felt that it was important to allay this anxiety. She did this by concentrating on the children. Everybody was interested in the children and the children's progress and care formed a "natural" topic of conversation and an obvious subject of the research.

Although she shared in the experience of caring for the children, the researcher also established her identity as a researcher. When she visited the Project, she always spent part of her time in the office looking at the children's records. This cut her off from the main activity in the bungalow. The researcher attended all staff and group meetings. The researcher clearly identified her role at these meetings as an observer and only made comments when invited to do so. Sometimes they wanted to use her as a source of expert advice so that they could use her information as a resource in the various debates and arguments in the Project. As far as possible she avoided being drawn into these arguments.

The researcher also established her role as a researcher by formally interviewing all the staff. Our first topic area was the recruitment and training of staff. The Research Director had monitored the selection process by attending the interviews and the researcher had monitored the training by attending the training sessions. To understand how trainers and trainees assessed the success of the training programme, the researcher carried out formal interviews with all the staff.

The first phase of the development of the relationship between the researcher and the Project staff lasted from August 1983 until November 1983 and was based on a balance. The researcher developed a relationship of reciprocity with the staff in the Project and used her normal social competence to achieve this (Crick, 1985, p.82). At the same time she engaged in defined research activities that differentiated and separated her.

The winter of 1983/4 was marked by a significant change in the Project. The Project settled into a pattern of routine operation and the initial excitement was replaced by a more realistic awareness of the scale of the tasks. Points of tension began to develop. As the winter came on so some staff were affected by ill health. As the atmosphere of the Project altered, so did the focus of the research. The staff in the Project still talked about the children but now they also wanted to talk about the management of the Project, the relationships in the Project and some of the frustrations of working in the Project. Some of the staff, especially the women, used the research worker as a confidante to whom they could express their fears and frustrations. The researcher, with her interest in feminism was willing and able to act as this confidante.

The shift in perspective was related to decisions made by the research team. The team had agreed to write an annual report on the overall progress of the Project and needed data on different aspects of the Project's operation. The shift was also a response to changing events in the Project.

In this stage of the research we continued to develop both our formal information gathering activities and informal relationship building. For example, the researcher conducted more formal interviews and had regular formal meetings with the Project Leader to discuss the progress of the Project and of the research. The research worker continued to talk to all the staff in the Project, and began to develop a closer and more intimate relationship with some of the staff in the style of ethnographic research (Griaule, 1965). Most of the care staff treated the researcher as a confidante, i.e. somebody outside the conflicts and tensions of the Project yet somebody who had sufficient knowledge to understand them and therefore to sympathise with their particular difficulties. However with some staff the relationship developed further. The researcher discussed her views and perspectives with them so that she could share her developing experience of the Project. She was exposing herself and her developing ideas.

There are costs of developing closer relations with informants, especially in situations of tension and conflict. It is easy to take sides and to understand the conflict from only one point of view. The researcher inevitably did take sides, she identified with and felt sympathy with the women workers. She had regular and informal contact with these women and allowed them to draw her into their world. On the other hand her relationship with the managers remained more formal. This relationship was changed by the third phase of the research, the preparation of research reports.

Writing Research Reports: Squaring the Circle of Informants, Gatekeepers and Sponsors

The production of research reports was a central part of our research process. We were conscious that as researchers we were taking information from our informants. Most researchers accept that it is good practice that the subjects of their research should be informed of the results of their research but usually this feedback is not seen as an integral part of the research process. Crick (1985) argued that researchers who used the ethnographic approach frequently made a radical shift in attitudes and role when they started writing their research reports. When they talked to their informant and recorded their activities and beliefs they identified with their informants. However, when they wrote their ethnographic texts they wrote "about" their informants. Johnson pointed out that very little is known about the impact of research publications on the people who provided the information. He suggested that informants should be involved in the production of research reports through a process of proof reading (Johnson, 1982, p.88). We wanted to do more than this. We wanted to involve our informants in the process of producing the accounts of their activities and beliefs.

We attached considerable importance to the early production of working papers and we decided to produce in the first year a paper on the process of staff selection and training. A final version was ready in April 1984. This draft was then distributed for comment to academic colleagues, to the care staff and to the managers in the Division. We provided individual copies and invited people to return these copies to us with comments. Our academic colleagues did this and their responses were generally favourable. None of the Barnardo's staff returned individual copies; instead the managers arranged special meetings to collate their views. The Project Leader organised these meetings and asked us not to attend as he felt it might inhibit discussion. The Project Leader then met the research worker to discuss the care staff's views. The response of the care staff was positive. They did not feel that the report was primarily addressed to them or criticised them. They felt it mainly concerned the managers who carried out the selection and the training. The care staff felt it provided them with an opportunity to comment on the training. We did not make any amendments to the report as a result of comments made by care staff.

The Divisional Director arranged a meeting of all senior staff and invited the Research Director and the researcher. The managers felt that the research team had failed to grasp their position as managers and as social workers. The meeting was an extremely unpleasant experience for us. We knew something had gone badly wrong. Some of the problems related to the structure of the first paper. These were relatively easy to rectify and we produced a revised paper. However we had also failed to take into account the managers' perspective and had failed to develop a close working relation with managers. We felt we would have to find ways of improving our relationship with managers and understanding their views.

When we redrafted the report and submitted it to the D.H.S.S. there were further problems. Their social work representatives were unhappy about some of the comments on social work practice. The D.H.S.S. were unhappy about the way in which we discussed the working paper with staff in Barnardo's before we submitted it to the Department.

The second working paper on the overall development of the Project in the first year was produced soon after the first working paper and there was no time to undertake a radical rethink of our strategy. In view of the D.H.S.S.'s concern about delays in receiving papers and the lack of individual response we had received from individual care staff, we decided not to provide each member of the care staff with a copy but made copies available to all managers and one for each bungalow.

Again, we got a little response from the care staff about this second paper. The care staff felt that the second working paper was more about them and their activities. Indeed there had been some anxiety amongst the care staff about the report. Some of the care staff found the paper long and difficult to read but they felt that it presented a realistic appraisal of the Project and their work in it. None of the care staff wanted any change. The response from senior staff was again more critical. They still felt that we did not really understand the importance of the social work context and the pressure under which they as managers had to operate.

The D.H.S.S. remained concerned about the process of handling papers. They felt that as they funded the research they should receive the working papers at the same time as Barnardo's. They felt that any prior discussion with Barnardo's could introduce bias. The Research Director explained that he felt that preliminary discussion with Barnardo's was an essential part of the research process. He acknowledged the D.H.S.S.'s concern about the delays this created but argued that these could be overcome through a speedier process of consultation. The D.H.S.S. did not pursue its objections.

As the main source of comment and criticism had come from divisional managers, we decided that care staff should receive copies of working papers after they were discussed with the divisional managers. Instead of arranging formal meetings with care staff to discuss the reports, the researcher discussed each paper informally. We established a regular monthly meeting with divisional managers. These arrangements made the process much faster.

We still felt that we needed to develop a greater awareness of the social work perspective and of the managers' perspective. We decided to seek the help of a social work colleague at the University. Heather Roughton agreed to act as a consultant to the project and to prepare material on social work issues.

When we started our research we focussed mainly on the Project. We underestimated the importance of the wider organisational context of the Project. It would have been useful in the original proposal to have included a study of the relationship between the Project and the Division. Our developing understanding of the importance of the divisional context was closely associated with our developing relationship with the Project Leader. In the first year of the research the Project Leader and the researcher had established a friendly and positive relation but it did not involve full trust and confidence. The researcher accepted that many of the criticisms made by the care staff could be explained by the structural position of the Project Leader but she also felt that some were a product of his style of management. The researcher felt that he sometimes avoided threatening issues by invoking professional or managerial confidence. The Project Leader felt that he could only discuss and explain part of his activities and his relations with staff in the Project. He felt that other matters were confidential, especially when they involved possible disciplinary issues or issues raised in supervision.

The problems came to a head in the summer of 1985 with the production of the second progress report on the Project. This report covered the period June 1984 to May 1985. It had been a particularly difficult period. The winter of 1984/5 was quite severe. Many staff were ill. Others left and there were inevitable delays in replacement. Staff felt under pressure and experienced a sense of crisis. Some felt that there was a contradiction between the normalisation philosophy and the realities of care. Our working paper reached the divisional managers at a particularly crucial time. The D.H.S.S. had told them that they were discussing the future funding of the Project and that the progress report would be taken into account in these discussions.

We had a very tense meeting with the divisional managers. However as a result of this meeting we developed a far better relationship with managers. We argued that our main source of information must be the care staff. The care staff had most contact with the children. They were also less powerful than managers and had less opportunity to change agency policy. However we accepted that managers were an equally important source of information and that it was important to regularly cross-check. The Project Leader also accepted the importance of open discussion with the research worker. He accepted that his classification of some information as confidential had deprived us of important information. He became more willing to discuss matters and the research worker no longer felt wary about raising issues with him. A relationship of greater confidence and trust developed based on perceptions of mutual benefit.

2.4 THE COSTS AND BENEFITS TO THE AGENCY

ALAN KENDALL AND GERRY DODSON

In the proposal to establish the Croxteth Park Project (then known as the Intensive Support Unit), we recognised the importance of having a research component linked to the project. Here are some of the things we said about it:

> In a project of this kind which is intended to demonstrate new possibilities for care and rehabilitation and so influence the direction of public policy, it is particularly important for a comprehensive evaluation to be carried out. Elements of such an evaluation might include
> (i) A cost/benefit analysis.
> (ii) A process evaluation of the systems developed by the project. It has often been noted in the past that children respond well to a transfer from large, hospital type institutions, to smaller, more "family-like" settings. However,

there is much less known about exactly what it is about the latter which leads to favourable changes.

That was sincerely meant. We felt that a new and innovative venture of this kind really needed to be carefully examined. It would be less than honest of us to acknowledge that we were looking for a sponsor and we felt that this would give added weight to the proposal itself. Moreover Barnardo's aims say that all our work is subject to evaluation and that we should be contributing to the development of child care knowledge and practice. However we did not anticipate that the research would take the form of a major project in its own right. When the D.H.S.S. offered to fund such research we welcomed it. Why shouldn't we? We were anxious to know how we were doing. We needed to know of our mistakes. Deep down we believed we would make a success of the Project, and so there was nothing really to bother about. And didn't we want to learn from our mistakes anyway? After all, we were professionals and this was the professional way of doing things. We had no idea what lay in store for us.

On the receiving end

We are social workers. We are not researchers. We approached this new project as social workers. What we wanted to do more than anything else was to give our children a good stimulating and caring home, and to show that our children could benefit from the sort of care we could offer, and that in fact they would develop better than they had done in their previous environments. We hoped, too, that we could go on to provide even better care for some of the children by placing them with substitute families. Now doing all that is a full-time job. We were very much in the risk business. Here we were taking children who were medically very problematic out of an environment that was felt, by many, to be essential for their needs. We were made aware, time and time again, of the very special needs of these children and young people, and the consequences that could arise from any inadequacy in the level of support to them. That made it a job and a half. And then on top of all that, we had this other major component - the research.

We were at the stage of interviewing for staff when the research project itself got under way. We had already appointed the Project Leader. The first real experience of "being researched" came when we were interviewing for residential social workers for the first phase of the project. Whilst we were interviewing candidates, commenting on them to one another, and coming to a decision, the Research Director scribbled furiously during the whole process. We were fascinated. What was he writing? What was he thinking? What was he making of us and the way we were going about things?

Well, if that was difficult, it was nothing compared to the first couple of reports we got from the research team. These were real eye openers to us. It was a shock to see things in print. To be quoted verbatim, swear words and all, was more than a little unnerving. Our comments and views were quoted. But did we really say that? Did we really mean that? Hadn't they got it out of context? And wasn't that little short of twisting what was said? Not only was it a shock to see things in print, but it was just as big a shock to realise that this was a foretaste of things to come. This was getting rather closer to us than we had anticipated. It was the first hint of the reality of research at Croxteth Park.

We had agreed with the research team that they would have every access to the Project's life and functioning, with two exceptions. These two things were the personnel records of members of staff and the notes of supervision sessions between the staff and their line managers. We felt that both of these items could contain quite personal information about an individual. Therefore confidentiality was our main concern and, although everything else was an open book, we took the view that staff were entitled to basic privacy. In real terms this meant that the researcher regularly attended staff meetings, group meetings, case conferences, reviews and staff development and training sessions within the Project. She could come and go as she pleased, having free access to every aspect of the daily life of the project. She was able to spend time there during any part of the day or night, during the week or weekends. She also had completely free access to all of the staff at the Project. She could observe them, converse with them, interview them or simply befriend whomsoever she chose.

Being on the receiving end of this type of research was, to say the least, very new for us all. Social workers are not accustomed to having their work observed in this way. In Croxteth Park, no matter what was going on at the time - from getting up in the mornings and having breakfast, throughout the day, during all the wide variety of activities, until bedtime - our actions were subject to scrutiny. Not only were Project staff affected, but this process also touched the children's parents, volunteers or anybody else visiting the Project. People would be seen talking amongst themselves, having fun, having a moan, feeling alert and feeling tired - they were always legitimate for the researcher.

Looking back now, it is hard to describe how that felt. There was a certain sense of being in a glass case or being under a microscope, a feeling which was to become quite average, almost to the point of acceptability. One wondered whether the dynamics of every situation were, in fact, influenced by the continual presence of this other person who was not a part of the Project itself, and who simply became absorbed into the daily culture of the Project. Now we knew what the Navajo Indians feel like with their families comprising mother, father, two children and a researcher. There were also, perhaps, particular pressures for people in line management positions, their roles and their actions were made much less anonymous. They could, and would be readily identifiable. This seemed to bring to some situations increased pressure, for example, when chairing meetings, there was always the feeling of being scrutinised, but in some particular situations, it felt like a test. Reactions were being watched, leadership assessed, and management skills appraised. Completely inaccurately, but perhaps quite naturally, there was a sense in the early stages of "They are looking to find fault", and for opportunities to be critical. This initial tension eased, but there was always a conscious awareness of an additional factor which could, in time, influence the future of our children and young people.

The first few months were quite difficult, especially for us as managers. The first two reports produced by the research team came as a great shock to us - as our reaction to the reports was to the researchers. To us as managers it seemed that the whole of the reports were biased towards the views, concerns, and work of the residential social workers. No account seemed to have been taken, or even the trouble to understand, the management and wider social work issues involved, let alone our views or difficulties. It seemed there was a danger of a chasm being created, with all the emphasis being in terms of the care staff. This could, in fact, have led to a reaction on the part of the management staff against care staff, let alone the research team. We had not expected, nor wanted, the research to be like this.

All this seems a long time ago now. Differences and difficulties were resolved. And we were all the better for it. We had to sit down with the research team and thrash the issues out. We had to understand their position and their concerns. We had to take on board the comments they were making, for some were indeed very valid and important. For their part, they had to understand the agency or management position. There were other valid and weighty points that needed to be taken account of. Managing residential services is a complex and difficult task. We felt they needed to understand that - and understand the reality of our position.

These initial difficulties lasted only a short period of time, and in the context of the whole of the research experience, were relatively unimportant. But it was very important in the sense that if the issues that were coming up then had not been addressed, had not been sorted out, and had not a constructive and friendly working arrangement come from it, the whole process would have been in grave danger.

The initial difficulties were sorted out in meetings between the senior divisional management staff responsible for Croxteth Park and Barnardo's Co-ordinator - Research and Development, and the research team. These first meetings led to a regular pattern of such discussions, which proved to be vital to the relationship. It would be hard to over-stress the importance of these regular meetings. Through them we have learned to trust and accommodate each other, for we could never agree on everything. We did develop a very close and fruitful working relationship in which we learned to acknowledge each other's position. This came about because both sides had the will to make it so. We both wanted it to work so there developed a flexibility on both sides. This was in no small part due to the attitude of the researchers which we came to know as one of sensitivity to our position, whilst at the same time maintaining their own independence and integrity. It is from those kinds of attitudes and approaches that trust grows.

We both needed that atmosphere of trust. For our part we knew we were making mistakes and would probably make more. Some of these we needed to have pointed out to us, but we also needed to be able to share them with the researchers in as open and frank a manner as possible. They certainly helped us to spot our mistakes and understand them. From this we were able to anticipate difficulties and indeed, in some instances, modify what we were doing.

Learning from the Research

The feedback from the research team came in three forms - day-to-day contact between the researcher and the Project Leader, written reports and the regular meetings.

As important as the meetings was the immediacy of the feedback on the research team's findings. Ongoing feedback came from the researcher to the Project Leader, and there was verbal feedback on a range of issues at the meetings we had with the research team. But mainly the feedback was through reports which were sent to us prior to our meetings. These were sent in draft and we were able to comment on them, correct any factual inaccuracies or misconceptions, but most of all - we were able to act. Having the findings in this way as soon as they were available turned out to be of great value to us. It would be hard to exaggerate this. There are three examples which will illustrate this.

We thought that the admission criteria contained in the original proposal were more than precise enough. However, this only served to indicate a difference in the thinking of social workers and researchers. The research team employed a far more precise and scientific definition of "profound mental handicap" against which they measured our first admissions. They also applied this in relation to prospective admissions following the placement of our children with families. Initially, we did not totally agree with them. We defined the "needs" of the children we were considering a little differently. The research team, through their criteria, were able to help us realise that there were wider issues at stake and the dangers we were running if we followed a more liberal admissions policy. The big danger lay in the possibility of opening ourselves up to the accusation that we were taking easier children, or children that it had already been shown could live outside the hospital setting. This was very important to us and we rethought our admissions policy and strictly adhered to their definition - i.e. that the child or young person should be functioning at less than six months.

The second example would be the procedure we followed during the induction of staff. Following the experience of the first group of staff to be selected and trained, it was clear from the research reports that we had not given enough time for the staff to spend with the children in hospital before their admission to Croxteth Park. The first group of staff felt they needed more time to gain confidence and skill in handling the children. We were able to adjust the second induction and training programme to allow for this.

A third example, and one that has had a considerable impact on the Division as a whole, related to the training of first line managers. The research team had highlighted weaknesses at first line manager level in Croxteth Park. We had been aware of these and had discussed them with the research team. We were able to identify areas requiring further training. We were also conscious that the needs of first line managers across the residential projects in the Division were similar to those at Croxteth Park. So we set up a divisional training programme for first line managers in all the residential projects in the division. This proved to be very successful, is ongoing, and places have recently been offered to other voluntary agencies in the area.

A point that should be made and appreciated by any manager who is involved with research work and research people is that there will be considerable demands on their time. The regular meetings (in our case about every two months) were time consuming in themselves, but the preparation for those meetings was even more time consuming than the meetings themselves. More often than not there were reports prepared by the researchers to discuss. These were often very lengthy. Moreover, because of the nature of things, the reports were often only available on the last minute. This may not seem a major issue. But we believe it is. To make the relationship work, and to get the best out of the research worker and the whole experience, demands a commitment from managers to invest in the process and give of their time.

Comment

As well as these specific examples, there are other benefits which we feel we have had from the presence of the research project. These have come from the ongoing interaction (of the relationship) with the research team over some five plus years. Their presence and feedback were used positively to motivate all of us to do better. The good results spurred us on. This was especially so when the information on the development of the children and young people began to come through. When you are very close to someone, it is sometimes difficult to really see objectively the progress that they are making. But there it was from the research team in black and white - irrefutable.

The constant presence of the researchers kept us on our toes. Having outsiders with different backgrounds and different perspectives examining and querying what was being done and why, makes you think, or rethink, things in a new way. Nothing can be taken for granted. Just because something had always been done in a particular way, or "everybody knows this is the way it should be" is no reason for continuing to do it. If we did we would never attempt anything new. Having someone who is interested in what you are doing, as the research team have been with us at Croxteth Park, is always a bonus. It was an interest, not just in the niceties of research, but we felt it was an interest in the project as a whole, and in our young people (and us).

Our experience of "being researched" has not always been an easy one. But nothing worthwhile is ever easy. The difficulties pale almost into insignificance against the positive experiences we have had. We believe that it has been a success and a joy. It is an experience we would have no hesitation in repeating. "Why?" you may ask. It can be narrowed down to two things. Firstly, we were very fortunate in the people we had working with us from the research team. We grew to trust and respect each other. And at times we had a lot of fun. Secondly, we had people in the research team who shared a similar vision to ourselves. People who, like us, really believed that together we had an opportunity to help, not only the children and young people at Croxteth Park, but hopefully countless others who we would never meet or never know.

2.5 SUMMARY AND COMMENT

Researchers using experimental or comparative approaches to evaluative research usually provide detailed accounts of their data collection procedures but often provide little information about the ways in which they developed relationships with the subjects of their research. Researchers using an ethnographic approach must provide detailed accounts of this relationship because it forms an essential part of their process of data collection.

In our research we had to develop and manage relations with our sponsors, the gatekeepers and our informants. Developing and managing these relations was not easy. At times we did not think we would succeed in maintaining honest, reciprocal relations with all the participants with their different and at times conflicting interests.

As researchers we feel that the ethnographic approach enabled us to collect detailed and rich data about the Project. However the approach is time consuming and, at times, emotionally demanding. It would not have been so successful if the staff and managers of Barnardo's had not been so sympathetic to research and so tolerant and patient. We were always able to discuss the issues openly and frankly and during the course of the research a positive and mutually beneficial relationship developed.

3 THE SELECTION AND TRANSFER OF THE CHILDREN

BIE NIO ONG AND ANDY ALASZEWSKI

We start the chapter with a general discussion of the process of inter-agency collaboration. We then describe and evaluate the process through which Barnardo's selected and transferred the children for the Croxteth Park Project.

3.1 INTER-AGENCY COLLABORATION

The policy of community care is now well established and there has been, over the last 30 years, a steady movement of mentally ill and mentally handicapped people from long-stay hospitals into the community. There have been few accounts of the process of selecting and transferring people, as most researchers have focussed on the planning process. For example, Korman and Glennerster (1985) have undertaken a major study of the transfer of mentally handicapped people from Darenth Park Hospital to community facilities. They concentrated on the planning process which was complex and "required a long process of bargaining during which the originally envisaged pattern of service changed significantly" (p.10). They suggested that the relationship was based on informal bargaining rather than rational joint planning. Korman and Glennerster found support for the closure of large long-stay hospitals and the development of alternative community-based facilities within both the NHS and local authorities. However there was considerable disagreement about the precise form of these alternative services and how they should be provided and funded (p.81).

There are some accounts of the early schemes to discharge patients from hospital to residential care in the community. These accounts tend to be very general (see Bodenham, 1983, Spencer, 1979, McKeown, 1980). One exception is a report by Haywood, Redmore and Ostle (1979) on the transfer of a unit for low-dependency mentally handicapped adults from the health service to social services. Although health service managers and social services officers agreed in principle that the hostel and its residents should be transferred, they had different perceptions of the residents' needs. The health professionals tended to see them as "patients" who required continual supervision and support whereas the social workers tended to view them as adults who needed housing and only a minimal level of support (pp.153-4). The final scheme was a compromise which was lubricated by joint finance money and created by pressure from senior managers in both agencies on the professionals involved in the negotiations.

The sensitive long-term care of highly dependent individuals such as profoundly mentally handicapped children requires the effective coordination of a range of welfare services, and in particular, health and social services. Any radical change in the pattern and balance of services, such as the closure of long-stay hospitals and the transfer of patients to community-based facilities is likely to create tensions between the various services. These tensions are related to the different structures and traditions of the services and to the different ways in which their staff perceive and respond to the needs of mentally handicapped people.

3.2 BARNARDO'S OBJECTIVES

In their application to the D.H.S.S., Barnardo's outlined the importance of demonstrating that profoundly handicapped children could be cared for outside mental handicap hospitals. Barnardo's wanted to select children for the project

> whose mental handicap is so profound, or so exacerbated by multiple physical handicaps, that they would not normally be considered for admission to any residential unit other than a mental handicap hospital. (Barnardo's, 1981c, p.4)

Barnardo's also specified that the children should be local, i.e. Liverpool based. They should be aged under 12 years on admission so that there was "sufficient time to work intensively

The Selection and the Transfer of the Children

with them and to plan for their future". They should not have behaviour problems that might endanger other more vulnerable children in the Project. They should not be suffering from a condition that would require in-patient treatment in an acute hospital, e.g. a malignant tumour, acute cardiac problems or a contagious disease.

Although these criteria appear straightforward, terms such as profound mental handicap have no clear or agreed meaning. To avoid confusion Barnardo's provided a more detailed definition of suitable children:

> The children will be displaying combinations of some of the following problems and conditions, in addition to mental handicap.
> (i)   Non-ambulant, often with varying degrees of paralysis.
> (ii) No speech, and little or no non-verbal communication.
> (iii) Sensory problems such as blindness or deafness.
> (iv) Double incontinence.
> (v)   Feeding problems.
> (vi) Epilepsy.
> (vii) Distortion of limbs and joints.
> (viii) Chronic respiratory problems. (Barnardo's, 1981c, p.6)

Barnardo's wanted to select eight children with profound handicaps and they wanted to maintain good relations with the hospitals providing the children. (For similar considerations in the Harperbury project see Shearer, 1981, p.21.) One manager described Barnardo's attitude to the health service in the following way:

> Building good relationships with the hospital was part and parcel of good practice and not a separate objective as such. We saw it as a method of achieving certain objectives; e.g. getting the children out of hospital. The children will require in-patient hospital care and in order to maintain the children in the Unit we need good working relationships with the hospital... We can't work in isolation and have to use the hospital when appropriate.

If the health workers had accepted Barnardo's objectives then co-operation would have been easy. However acceptance of the Project varied. The hospital social workers were the most enthusiastic supporters of the Project as they saw it as a means of deinstitutionalising children. Senior staff were unsure. The

Project would be an important resource local resource if it worked. More junior staff, especially ward nurses, tended to see the Project as a competitor. Nurses stressed the importance of the emotional ties that they had developed with the children:

> It's like you having a child and rearing it and then have somebody come along and say to you "Oh well we're going to take them away, we think someone else can do better than you, and we are going to take him off you".

Despite the perceived threat to jobs in the hospital, all the hospital staff supported both the general principle of community care and the establishment of residential units in ordinary houses in the community. However there was little support amongst ward nurses for moving profoundly handicapped children. Ward nurses wanted to discharge the *most able* children first as they felt that these children would benefit most from living in units such as the Croxteth Park Project.

Comment

The main objective of the senior Barnardo's personnel for the selection was clear-cut. They wanted profoundly and/or multiply handicapped children. They needed the co-operation of the health service to identify the initial group of children, to minimise the disruption that these children might experience when transferred, and to maintain a high standard of health care for children after the move.

If there had been total support in the health service for the Project and its objectives, then Barnardo's would have experienced no tension between its concern to select profoundly and/or multiply mentally handicapped children and its desire to maintain good relations with the N.H.S. Senior managers and practitioners in the N.H.S. could see the Project as an important local resource but ward staff tended to view the Project as a threat. This tension did not manifest itself in a direct rejection of the principles of community care and the Project, but rather, manifested itself in disagreements about the suitability of specific children.

3.3 THE PROCESS OF SELECTING AND TRANSFERRING THE CHILDREN

The selection involved the senior Barnardo's personnel and their professional advisors and the majority of the negotiations took place with senior hospital personnel. The actual transfer of the children took place rather later, after the Project staff had been selected and after the bungalows had been furnished and decorated. The transfer also involved senior staff in both Agencies but they played more of an enabling role. The front line care staff, the ward nurses and the R.S.W.s had to work together to prepare the children for transfer to the Project.

The Process of Selecting the Children

The main decisions were made by a working party consisting of managers and professional staff of the North West Division. This working party was responsible for managing the establishment of the Project until the appointment of the Project Leader in March 1983 (see Table 3.1 for overall timetable). There were two key elements in the selection process; collecting and assessing information about possible children in local hospitals and assessing parental attitudes to the transfer.

Collecting and Assessing Information Senior personnel in Barnardo's were conscious of the fact that many of the children in the Project would have health problems and would, on occasion, require urgent treatment. They had to be sure that the staff of the Project could provide or obtain the necessary treatment. Therefore the working group needed accurate information about the needs of the children and the type of care R.S.W.s could provide. Much of this information on the children would have to come from hospital staff. Although hospital staff did not try to mislead Barnardo's, they tended to stress the medical fragility of the children, their recurrent health problems and the difficulties of providing nursing and medical care. The senior personnel needed expert advice to get a realistic appraisal of the problems and risks involved. For this advice they used their own psychologists and medical adviser.

Before the initial meeting of the working party, Barnardo's own psychologists visited the local hospitals and identified 14 children who might be suitable for the Project. At the initial meeting of the working party the psychologists gave a preliminary assessment of the 14 children. The working party discussed the medical needs and conditions of the children. The working party decided to select 8 children for admission and also to have a reserve list. They agreed that the "criteria should be used flexibly."

Table 3.1
Timetable of Main Events Associated with Transfer of the Children from Hospital to the Croxteth Park Project

1979	Initial proposal by Divisional Director for the establishment of the Project.
1980	Application to D.H.S.S. for a grant to establish the Project, initial contact with hospitals.
Feb. 1981	D.H.S.S. agrees a grant for the Project.
Oct. 1982	Working group established to set up the Project.
Nov. 1982	Detailed collection of information about the children and initial discussion in working group. Initial list of 13 children.
Dec. 1982	Discussion with Barnardo's medical consultant at about the medical and nursing needs of the children. Final selection of children for Phase 1, Phase 2 and reserve list.
Jan. 1983	Stuart seriously ill and withdrawn from list for Phase 1 and replaced by Ivan.
Feb. 1983	Jimmy's parents refuse permission for Jimmy's transfer. Jimmy withdrawn from Phase 1 and replaced by Connie.
Mar. 1983	Project Leader appointed.
June 1983	R.S.W.s for Phase 1 start training programme.
July 1983	Barnardo's informed by hospital that Gillian could not come and that she would be replaced by Rob. Barbara and David admitted to Phase 1.
Aug. 1983	Connie and Rob admitted to the first Phase. Training of R.S.W.s for Phase 2 starts.
Dec. 1983	Mark, Margaret, Linda and Ivan admitted to Phase 2.

The Selection and the Transfer of the Children

The psychologists were asked to assess the children and to compile a shortlist.

At the next meeting (end of November) the psychologists had completed their assessment of 13 children (one had been fostered). The working party accepted the psychologists' view that children requiring special medical treatments such as the rectal administration of valium, should not be considered for the first phase of the Project but might be considered for the second phase, when the Project staff had more experience. This reduced the shortlist to 7 children (see Table 3.2).

Table 3.2
Shortlist of Children for the First Phase
(Nov. 1982)

Hillside Hospital	Jimmy	Aged	4
	Mark	Aged	6
	Gillian	Aged	12
Plum Hill Hospital	David	Aged	9
	Ivan	Aged	10
	Margaret	Aged	12
Raventree Hospital	Andrew	Aged	8

To be sure that the R.S.W.s could care for these children, the working party consulted Barnardo's medical adviser. The medical adviser felt that the R.S.W.s should be able to cater for all the normal care needs of the children selected for the first phase. However he felt that some of the children might not be handicapped enough to fit the original criteria and that the working party might consider admitting more severely handicapped children. The medical adviser discussed the medical needs of the children and the extent to which R.S.W.s would be able to perform different care procedures, i.e. the use of suction to clear fluid from the children's lungs, intravenous injection of valium, the rectal administration of valium, tube feeding and physiotherapy. He was able to reassure the working party that R.S.W.s should be able to perform all these treatments except for intravenous injection of valium. He suggested Barnardo's should see if valium could be administered rectally rather than intravenously. In the light of this advice the working party decided to reconsider all the children.

The Selection and the Transfer of the Children

Two of the 13 children were excluded because they were acutely ill. The remaining children were considered handicapped enough to require placement in the Project but medically sound enough to benefit (see Table 3.3).

Table 3.3
Selection (Dec. 1983)

Hillside Hospital

Jimmy	aged 4	Phase 1
Connie	aged 4	Reserve List, Intravenous valium
Linda	aged 4	Phase 2
Mark	aged 6	Phase 2
Joanna	aged 12	Not listed - tube fed and too ill to attend school
Gillian	aged 12	Phase 1

Plum Hill Hospital

Barbara	aged 8	Phase 1
David	aged 9	Phase 1
Sean	aged 9	Not listed - chest condition
Ivan	aged 10	Reserve list, not local
Stuart	aged 10	Phase 2
Margaret	aged 12	Phase 2

Raventree Hospital

| Andrew | aged 8 | Reserve list, possibly too able |

One child, Connie, was placed on the reserve list because she was prescribed intravenous valium but the working party decided to ask her consultant if her valium could be administered rectally. Andrew was placed on the reserve list because he was the most able child to be considered and it was possible that an alternative placement would be found for him. Ivan was placed on the reserve list. He was not local and his admission was considered less urgent as he was receiving additional support from respite foster parents.

Jimmy and David were allocated to the first phase and the working party decided to allocate Barbara and Gillian to this phase as they felt that they were two of the most profoundly handicapped children. Mark and Margaret were then allocated to the second phase together with Linda and Stuart (See Table 3.3).

At the beginning of January 1983 the psychologist, while visiting the hospital, discovered that Stuart's medical condition had suddenly deteriorated and he was being treated in an oxygen tent. Barnardo's felt that Stuart was no longer suitable for admission to the unit as he was in the acute phase of an illness. Following consultations with the Barnardo's medical adviser, Ivan was substituted for Stuart.

Discussing the Transfer with Parents

In mid-January the psychologist wrote to the hospital social workers at Plum Hill Hospital and Hillside Hospital confirming the names of the children that had been selected for the Project. At Plum Hill Hospital there were no problems about visiting the parents. The contact with the parents of the children at Plum Hill Hospital, i.e. David's and Barbara's parents, went smoothly. They were visited by a psychologist from Barnardo's and the hospital social worker and agreed to the transfer of their children.

However, at Hillside Hospital there were problems. The hospital team decided that the medical staff should speak to the parents first. In February Gillian's and Jimmy's parents had an interview with the hospital consultants and agreed to the transfer of their children and to meeting a representative from Barnardo's. However, before the hospital social worker and a Barnardo's representative could visit Jimmy's parents they changed their minds and decided that they did not want him to be transferred. The reasons for their decision were never made clear to Barnardo's. When the hospital social worker heard about Jimmy's parents' decision, she decided to offer a place in the first phase to Connie who was on the reserve list for the Project. Barnardo's had been unwilling to accept her because she had been prescribed intravenous valium if and when she had an epileptic fit. As her prescription had been changed to rectal valium, Barnardo's were willing to accept her for the first phase.

The Selection and the Transfer of the Children

There was one very late change. One of the consultants in Liverpool was responsible for the care of a young multiply handicapped child. Rob was 3 years old and was in Hillside Hospital. His parents appeared to have rejected him. Both the consultant and the ward nurses felt that his placement in hospital was unsuitable and that he should be discharged as quickly as possible. When the psychologist was assessing Connie in hospital in January 1983, the nurses drew her attention to Rob. She said that Barnardo's might be willing to consider him in the future. In March the hospital social worker asked Barnardo's to accept Rob. At the same time the hospital consultant discussed Rob's future with his parents and they agreed to allow him to be discharged from hospital. In July 1983 Barnardo's were informed by the hospital that Rob was replacing Gillian. Rob had not been assessed and it was not clear that he fell within the criteria for admission to the Project. Rob's consultant had offered Rob's parents a place in the Project. Barnardo's felt that they could not let the parents down. Furthermore, Rob's consultant was willing to become the medical consultant for all the children in the Project and this would solve the problem of access to specialist facilities. Barnardo's therefore decided to carry out an assessment of Rob. This assessment indicated that Rob did fit the criteria for admission. Barnardo's therefore decided to accept him.

The Transfer of the Children

The senior personnel in Barnardo's attached considerable importance to ensuring a smooth transfer of the children from the hospital to the Project. They were conscious that transfers often take place abruptly with little preparation of either staff or the children. They wanted to reduce this abruptness by making the transfer of children a more gradual process. Therefore, they built the process of the transfer into the training programme for the care staff.

The training programme included a period of work in the hospitals. In the original training programme this period was not specified but it was clearly envisaged as a fairly short period. The ward staff were initially informed by senior hospital staff that the R.S.W.s would work in the hospital for about three days to get to know the children. The ward staff felt that this was far too short. Following discussions with the hospital staff, the Project Leader agreed that the R.S.W.s should spend two weeks working with the

The Selection and the Transfer of the Children

children on the ward. The R.S.W.s from Phase One who worked in Plum Hill spent two weeks on the wards. The R.S.W.s from Phase One who worked in Hillside Hospital worked for about four weeks on the wards. This was partly the result of the late substitution of Rob for Gillian. The R.S.W.s in the second phase planned to spend four weeks on the ward and eventually spent 8 weeks on the wards. During their period in hospital the R.S.W.s worked alongside the nursing staff getting to know the children, identifying their needs and gaining experience in caring for them.

Comment

The senior personnel in the North West Division were very conscious that the Project was experimental and that their decisions and actions would be subject to scrutiny. Getting the "right" children was vital. They also had to be sure that they did not select any children who the R.S.W.s could not care for. As the Project represented a new model of care the working group was cautious and careful about the selection of the children. They relied heavily on their professional advisers to collect information and to provide them with advice and guidance.

At Plum Hill Hospital the transfer of the children went relatively smoothly. At Hillside Hospital there were repeated problems. Neither of the two children selected for first Phase was actually transferred. The precise reasons for these problems were unclear, but seemed to be related to the internal problems and tensions of the hospital, i.e. it was scheduled for closure, and to a basic disagreement between hospital staff and Barnardo's about the sort of children that should be transferred to the Project.

3.5. ASSESSING THE PROCESS

In this section we shall first provide an assessment of the children's suitability for the Project based on our psychological assessments. We shall then provide subjective evaluations of the transfer based on the perceptions of staff in Barnardo's and of the hospital staff.

Psychological Assessment of the Children

In his first psychology report, Steven Lovett assessed the

The Selection and the Transfer of the Children

suitability of the first 8 children admitted to the Project. He used a strict definition of profound handicap. For the purposes of his assessment a profoundly handicapped child should not perform at above the 6 month development level nor exhibit any forms of behaviour associated with older children, e.g. mobility or speech. As there is no single test standardised on profoundly mentally handicapped children, he used three separate tests and we shall report the results of each test.

The Bayley Scale of Infant Development Generally the children were performing at a fairly low level on the Bayley Scale. Most of the children were performing at a mental age level of between 2 months and 6 months although their motor age was slightly higher, 2 months to 9 months. The children's performance tended to be inconsistent. They often failed relatively easy items yet passed more difficult ones. This variation is typical of the performance of profoundly handicapped children and has been reported in other studies (Sebba, 1978). On the mental age scale the most consistent performers were Mark and David and the least consistent, Margaret, Linda and Rob. On the motor scale the most consistent performers were Mark and Ivan and the least consistent, Margaret and Linda. It appears that the more able children had the wider scatter of performances.

Physically (i.e. motor age), the most advanced children were Connie (6.5 months), Margaret (6.0 months) and Linda (9.0 months). The lower performance of Rob on the motor age scale when compared to a mental age scale was related to his physical handicaps. There was a clear rank ordering when the categories in which children scored over 50% were examined.

Mark	- over 50% in 1 category
Ivan	- over 50% in 1 category
Barbara	- over 50% in 2 categories
David	- over 50% in 3 categories
Rob	- over 50% in 5 categories
Connie	- over 50% in 6 categories
Margaret	- over 50% in 10 categories
Linda	- over 50% in 12 categories

In general all the children showed a lack of responsiveness to the test items on the Bayley Scale. This would be expected with a group of profoundly handicapped children. Only Rob, Margaret and Linda seemed to be performing at a more advanced level.

The Object Schemes Scale assesses the way in which a child interacts with objects in his or her environment. The behavioural schemes are organised in a hierarchy starting at the two months level with the mouthing of objects and progressing to the 18 months level with the naming of objects. As with the Bayley Scale there was an uneven performance. Only four of the 8 children mouthed objects, a behaviour that would be expected in a normal three month old baby. On the other hand 5 children dropped three or more objects, a behaviour that would be expected in an 8-9 month old child.

Mark and Ivan did not interact at all with the objects. Connie and Barbara interacted with the objects in a way that would be expected of a four month old baby. David, Rob, Margaret and Linda had higher levels of performance and interacted with the objects in a way that one would expect of a child between 6 and 9 months old.

The Behavioural Assessment Battery does not provide a global score; rather it provides an indication of the strengths and weaknesses of the children in different areas of performance.

All the children exhibited some ability to interact with their environment. For example, all the children except Mark and Barbara passed over 50% of the items assessed on the auditory skills. However the children did not do as well on the items which assessed more sophisticated types of interaction with their environment. For example, only Linda and Rob passed 50% of the tracking skill items and only Linda and Rob scored over 50% on the inspection skills. On the social skills all the children passed some of the items. Indeed given the extent of the children's handicap it was somewhat surprising to find that all the children manifested some self-help skills, albeit none passed more than 10% of the self-help items. Generally there was a smaller variation in performance on these items. Linda, Rob and Margaret tended to perform at a higher level than the other children. All the children, except Ivan, exhibited some form of exploratory play but only Rob exhibited any form of constructive play and search strategies. Only Rob, Connie and surprisingly Ivan, exhibited any form of perceptual problem solving.

Comment

As a group the children exhibited many of the characteristics of profoundly handicapped children. Not only was their performance low but it was also extremely variable. Two of the children, Mark and Ivan, were extremely handicapped and on the Object Scheme Scale exhibited no established schemes of behaviour. Margaret, Linda and Rob were performing at higher levels than the other children. There was a third group of children, Connie, Barbara and David whose performance was between the two extremes. These children had some variable performances. For example, Connie performed at a relatively high level in the motor part of the Bayley Scale and David performed well in the Object Scheme Scale. Mark, Ivan, Connie, Barbara and David were clearly profoundly mentally handicapped children. Margaret, Linda and Rob were undoubtedly severely handicapped but their suitability for the Project requires further consideration.

Margaret was both profoundly and multiply mentally handicapped, but did possess a relatively high level of interactive skills when relating to her environment. The results of the Bayley Scale and the Behavioural Assessment Battery indicated that she was functioning at the higher end of the profound mental handicap range. She had some speech, although it was difficult to assess the extent to which she used words purposively. At the time of her admission she was probably suitable for the Project, especially if her multiple health problems were taken into account.

Linda was not profoundly or multiply mentally handicapped in a strict definition of these terms. She was clearly very responsive to her environment and acted upon it adaptively. Linda was mentally handicapped, had physical problems and was profoundly deaf. The education authority identified her main handicap as one of hearing loss and she attended a school for the deaf.

Rob was not profoundly and multiply mentally handicapped. He had no visual or hearing handicaps. He was however, profoundly physically handicapped through cerebral palsy caused by lack of oxygen at birth. He may have had some residual mental handicap but this was extremely difficult to detect or assess in such a young child.

Barnardo's Assessment

Overall Barnardo's were happy with the outcome of both the selection and transfer of the children although there were aspects

The Selection and the Transfer of the Children

of both processes that they felt could have been improved. Only four of the 8 children initially admitted to the Project fully fitted the "strict" criteria but 7 were suitable in terms of handicap (see Table 3.4). The senior personnel at Barnardo's felt that the criteria were guidelines rather than a rigid set of rules. They felt that it was important that all the children were profoundly handicapped.

Table 3.4
Suitability of the Children Admitted According to Senior Personnel

Child	Profound Mental Handicap	Age (Under 12)	Liverpool Based Placement	Suitable for Project
Mark	Yes	Yes	Yes	Yes
Ivan	Yes	Yes	No	Yes
Connie	Yes	Yes	Yes	Yes
Barbara	Yes	Yes	Yes	Yes
David	Yes	Yes	Yes	Yes
Margaret	Yes	No	Yes	Yes
Linda	Yes	Yes	No	Yes
Rob	Possibly	Yes	No	Possibly

They did not feel that age or place of birth was as important. For example Margaret was just over age when she was admitted to the Project. The senior personnel felt that Margaret was the sort of child that the Project was designed for and that she would benefit from placement in the Project.

Although the senior personnel in Barnardo's were happy about the outcome of the selection procedure, they were less happy about some aspects of the process, in particular they felt that Connie's and Rob's selection did not follow the correct procedure. In neither case were they consulted about the child. In Rob's case the problems were serious. Barnardo's felt that they had been subjected to severe pressure. If they refused Rob, they would have seriously damaged their relationship with the consultant and it would have been very traumatic for Rob's parents. They felt that in the circumstances they had little choice.

The Selection and the Transfer of the Children

The divisional managers felt that the transfer of the children from the hospital to the Project went well. They felt that none of the children had been damaged by the process and that the R.S.W.s had been able to build up their confidence in their ability to care for their children and to build on the experience and knowledge of hospital staff. They felt that the R.S.W.s who had worked longest in hospital had gained most. The senior personnel did acknowledge that there were problems. They felt that some of these problems were due to miscommunication within the hospitals. For example, they felt that staff in Hillside Hospital had been misinformed about the length of time the transfer would take place.

The front-line staff were not involved in the negotiations about the selection of the children. They were, however, closely involved in and they did have strong views about the transfer of the children.

The first group of R.S.W.s felt their relationship with the hospital staff was very difficult and that nurses, particularly in Hillside Hospital, were reluctant to let their children go. They did not feel it was entirely the hospital's fault. Some felt Barnardo's had contributed to the problem through inadequate preparation. The first group of R.S.W.s found their work in hospital very difficult but recognised that it was very important.

The R.S.W.s from the second phase learnt from the experiences of Phase One and established far better working relations with the ward staff. Although they felt the transitional period was long, they felt they had received considerable support from ward staff.

Assessment by the Hospital Staff

The ward staff in the hospital acknowledged the importance of discharging mentally handicapped children into a community-based facility but they felt that the least handicapped children should be discharged first. There was some concern amongst the ward staff about the ability of the Project to provide the necessary nursing care for the children and in particular the extent to which the Project could provide specialist support services such as medical advice or physiotherapy. However their main concern was the suitability of the children. Many of the ward staff felt that some of the children selected for the Project were so severely handicapped that they could not be expected to improve and that money was being wasted on such handicapped children and could be better used on less severely handicapped children. Therefore they felt that only the three most able children were suitable (see Table 3.5).

Table 3.5
Suitability of the Children Admitted According to Hospital Ward Nursing Staff

	Needs for Nursing	Needs Physio-therapy	Has Developmental Potential	Has Sufficient Awareness	Suitable for the Project
Mark	No	No	No	No	No
Ivan	No	Yes	No	No	No
Connie	Yes	No	No	No	No
Barbara	No	Yes	No	No	No
David	No	Yes	No	No	No
Margaret	Yes	Yes	Yes	Yes	Yes
Linda	Sometimes	No	Yes	Yes	Yes
Rob	No	No	Yes	Yes	Yes

The nurses in the hospital had clear views about the process of selection. Nursing managers felt that Barnardo's had not recognised the importance of nurses in the decision-making process. Barnardo's had approached the doctors and then made contact with the hospital social workers who asked ward staff to draw up a list of all children under 12 years old from the Liverpool area. The nurse managers did not feel that the purpose of this exercise had been properly explained to them. Furthermore they felt that Barnardo's had altered their criteria for selection. However, they did accept that were problems in the hospitals.

At Plum Hill Hospital the ward nurses did not feel threatened by the selection process. They felt that the process had been a collaborative one between the ward sisters and the hospital social worker. In Hillside Hospital the tensions were far greater. The ward sisters felt that they had had little input into the selection procedure and had not been sufficiently consulted.

Generally nurses felt that the transition period was important and was an essential part of establishing the Project. The nurses felt that the longer period that the Phase Two R.S.W.s had spent in the hospital had been of great benefit for their preparation. The nurses felt that they had given the R.S.W.s a good start.

Comment

The transfer of patients from the health service to social work agencies such as Barnardo's is bound to be a difficult and at times tense process. The agencies have different cultures, operate in different ways and have different traditions and work practices. It is difficult to overcome professional rivalries and professional distrust. The staff in the hospital may feel their past contribution is being devalued. Korman and Glennerster (1985) described a similar process in Darenth Park Project:

> Darenth was left out, excluded from the exciting new developments. Staff who had worked many years in large institutions were thought to have little to offer a new style of service. (p.147)

The discharge of mentally handicapped children from hospital can be a traumatic and emotional experience for the nurses. The children discharged to the Project were very vulnerable. In many cases they had been in hospital since they had been babies and they had depended on the care and affection of the nurses. In many cases the nurses had grown attached to the children. It was inevitable that they would experience some jealousy of the Project and see its establishment as an implicit criticism of their ability to care for the children.

3.4 SUMMARY AND COMMENT

To overcome the inevitable fears and apprehensions of the nurses and to reassure them, the process of selection and transfer of the children required sensitive and skilful management. The ward staff needed information about the Project, the sort of children Barnardo's wanted and the type of care they would provide for these children. Ward staff did not receive this information until late in the process. In many cases they received it from the R.S.W.s. There were a variety of reasons for these difficulties.

The process of selecting the children was managed by a

The Selection and the Transfer of the Children

working party of divisional managers and professional advisors. The Project Leader was not appointed until relatively late in the process. All the members of the working party had other commitments. This meant that no single person in the Division was in a position to take on full-time responsibility for negotiating with the hospitals and ensuring the right information was given to ward staff. The psychologists did play a leading role in establishing contact with the hospital but they did not have the time or the expertise of a Project Leader.

Barnardo's decided to use the hospital social workers as their main avenue of contact with the hospital. As Barnardo's is a social work agency and the hospital social workers were sympathetic to the objectives of the Project this was a reasonable decision. However it did create difficulties. The hospital social workers were not part of the main hospital culture and probably found it difficult to understand the anxieties and concerns of nurses. Barnardo's probably did not allow for the hierarchical nature of the hospitals. Information given to hospital social workers, consultants or senior nurse managers did not reach ward nurses. Barnardo's were understandably reluctant to interfere in the internal management of the hospitals. However, earlier and more direct contact with the ward staff to explain the objectives of the Project and the apparent changes in guidelines might have allayed some of the fears and anxieties.

The senior divisional managers wanted to reduce the abruptness of the transfer of responsibility of care from the ward staff to the R.S.W.s. The period of work in the hospitals was a major innovation. It generally seemed to improve relations between the Project and the hospitals and enabled the R.S.W.s to gain confidence in their ability to care for the children and to learn from the experiences of the ward nurses. However there were costs. Young and relatively inexperienced R.S.W.s were placed in an environment in which they sometimes felt threatened and isolated. Most of them did not enjoy the experience but they did feel it was essential and that they had gained a lot from it.

4 THE SELECTION AND TRAINING OF THE STAFF

BIE NIO ONG AND ANDY ALASZEWSKI

We start this chapter with a general discussion of the process of selecting and training staff for community units. We then describe and evaluate the process through which Barnardo's selected and trained staff for the Project.

4.1 SELECTING AND TRAINING THE STAFF

The shift from care in institutions to care in the community involves more than a change in the physical location of care. It involves a major change in skills and attitudes. Institutions were not just places in which people with a mental handicap were cared for, they were also places in which staff acquired attitudes and skills for care. The shift towards care in the community requires not only a new set of attitudes and skills but also a new mechanism for creating them.

The concern with staff and training has formed a major theme within policy documents. Policy-makers accept that it is important to increase the supply of suitably qualified professionals. However, progress "establishing a common framework for statutory training relevant to the community-based residential services" has been slow (Towell, 1983, p.54). Care staff without formal training will continue to provide the bulk of residential care (Welsh Office, 1983, p.31). If the new community-based residential services are to avoid the pitfalls of the old institutions then special attention has to be devoted to the recruitment and training of care staff.

New community-based units do not fit neatly into the existing structures of service agencies. Recruiting staff to the new community units is difficult and time consuming because there are often no ground rules. Existing job descriptions and formal qualifications are inappropriate because the new units are so different from the large institutions which they are replacing (Ward, 1984a, p.17).

Senior managers in local health and social service agencies are beginning to grapple with the problems of recruiting and training staff for the new community-based units. A number of the early schemes have been documented and certain common problems and issues can be identified. All reports stress the importance of selecting the "right" staff (Abbott and Chamberlain, 1986, p.51) but it is difficult to define "right". The King's Fund working party stressed the importance of identifying the skills required rather than assuming individuals with a formal qualification would have such skills (Towell, 1980, p.33). The working party responsible for establishing the Bolton Neighbourhood Network Scheme (1984) were also concerned about the limitations of formal qualifications.

Many projects have thought long and hard about the type of staff which they are trying to attract. A major dilemma here has been the choice between health service and social service personnel. Some projects have decided that health service personnel would not be appropriate for the new facilities as they would be in danger of bringing "institutional" ideas to the new model of care. Others value the wealth of experience that health service staff possess and believe that they are an important resource which should be developed (PSSRU, 1985). In the Wells Road Service in Bristol, the managers used administrative/clerical grades rather than nursing grades so that the unit could recruit people from a wide circle of backgrounds. Applicants *without* formal training or even relevant experience were often just as suitable as those with more traditional qualifications and experience (Ward, 1984a, p.39).

As formal qualifications and experience cannot be used as a guide for selecting staff, managers have to develop their own criteria for selection. Ward identified a number of possible criteria. Broadly these can be divided into three groups:

> * personal characteristics, e.g. warm personality, interpersonal skills, flexibility and initiative
> * ideological commitment, e.g. interest in, and apparent commitment to, the ideas behind the new service (normalisation etc.)

> * team compatibility, e.g. mix of personalities, with quieter staff to complement more outgoing members.

Ward (1984a) placed very little emphasis on experience and skills. Indeed they only appeared in her list as part of the team compatibility criteria.

In the literature, there are discussions of the sort of people who should be selected to staff the new community units and there is some agreement about the criteria that should be used to select these people. However, there is far less discussion of the process by which these people should be selected. The selection process tends to be discussed in terms of conventional activities such as advertising, shortlisting and interviewing. For example, Ward saw contact between applicants and any existing staff in the unit as an optional part of the process (Ward, 1984a, p.38).

The emphasis on personal qualities rather than formal qualifications in the selection process means that staff with varying levels of experience and qualifications are being recruited to community units. They require training to prepare them for their responsibilities. A commitment to staff training can be seen in all the Care in the Community schemes monitored by the Personal Social Services Research Unit at Kent University. All the projects listed some training activities and in the majority of cases this involved induction training courses (PSSRU, 1987, pp. 16-23).

Traditionally training courses have concentrated on developing the care skills of staff. This element is present in the training courses for new units (See Allen, 1983, pp. 35-37). However there is also a wider concern. The training is usually designed to build teams and develop the right attitudes.

These wider training objectives are associated with the use of progressive training techniques. Traditional class-based learning is minimised and interactive group learning is stressed. Allen described the approach to "team building" in the Northumberland scheme in the following way:

> In part this was people-oriented - concentrating on developing a climate of trust and openness in which members of the group could respond to each other's professional and personal needs, in which enthusiasm was encouraged and in which conflict - within limits - was seen as creative. In part it was task-oriented - making use of individual strengths, teaching necessary skills and helping

staff use time well. They learned to balance the two approaches and why both were important to the life of the team. (Allen, 1983, p.38)

Raynes and Sumpton have approached the training issue from a different angle. They asked community staff what type of training they would like. Care staff did perceive a need for training and Raynes and Sumpton grouped these perceived needs in 17 areas. Care staff wanted information about and training in ideology, team/social skills and personal skills but they also wanted more traditional forms of training and information:

> All groups perceived a need for training in basic knowledge of the causes - social, psychological, and medical - of mental handicap. At all levels staff asked for training in ways of dealing with difficult behaviour and in basic skills such as lifting, dealing with incontinence, and counselling of residents. (Raynes and Sumpton, 1987, p.96)

Comment

Caring for mentally handicapped people in the community is demanding and staff trained and experienced in caring for mentally handicapped people in an institutional setting may not have the "right" skills and attitudes. As the current system of formal training is not seen as appropriate and there are no immediate prospects of an alternative formal system of training, managers setting up a unit must establish their own criteria for selecting staff and must establish their own systems of training to ensure that staff have the necessary skills and attitudes.

Managers tend to use traditional methods of recruiting staff, e.g. advertising and interviewing, but they do not use traditional criteria. Formal qualifications and previous experience, especially nursing qualifications and experience of caring for mentally handicapped people in hospitals, are regarded with some suspicion and instead selectors emphasise the importance of personal characteristics such as the right attitude and an ability to fit into a team.

There is a similar change in attitudes to training. In an institutional setting training has traditionally been limited to a relatively small group of staff undertaking professional courses. In community units *all* staff are seen as needing substantial preparation and training. There is also a shift in methods. The preparation of staff for work in the community unit is seen as a far more complex process. It is more than providing skills and knowledge. It is also about changing attitudes and building teams. Traditional class-based teaching must be supplemented by more interactive styles of learning.

4.2 OBJECTIVES OF BARNARDO'S FOR SELECTION AND TRAINING OF CARE STAFF

Barnardo's places emphasis on the development of individual members of the agency through training and supervision and through their involvement in innovatory schemes. A commitment to service development is associated with a commitment to staff development. To be a successful service development the Croxteth Park Project has not only to recruit personnel but also to train them.

There was, in the Project, a blurring of the distinction between staff selection, training and management. Senior personnel saw staff selection, training and management as part of the same process of getting the "right" staff with the "right" attitudes and skills to care for the children in the "right" way. "Right" was defined by senior personnel of the agency and in terms of the principles of normalisation. Senior personnel felt that the staff were crucial to the success of the project:

> When it comes down to it no matter what resources there are, the most important resource is people. You need people who believe that they can bring about change... We need people who believe our children are special and will do wonderful things. And when they believe that, wonderful things do happen.

Objectives in the Selection of R.S.W.s

One senior manager described the criteria for staff selection in the following way:

> What we wanted for the Unit were people who were prepared to work together as a team, had very similar attitudes to the children in their relationships and ability to develop, could agree with the concept that children should not live in hospital, could value children, had enthusiasm, had belief

and energy.

The concern with the right attitudes was a main theme in the selection of R.S.W.s. Some of the interviewers felt that attitudes once formed were difficult, if not impossible to change. As the Project was innovative, experience in routine and traditional services was seen as a possible problem. The selection panel were concerned not only with under-commitment but also with over-commitment, e.g. they were not sure that individuals with their own mentally handicapped children would make good R.S.W.s.

The interview panel was also concerned to assess the extent to which any particular applicant could work with other staff in the unit and fit into a team. The panel was concerned about individuals who had different backgrounds to the majority of the applicants. The interview panel were more interested in the general social skills of the applicants than their specific technical skills.

Divisional managers' concern with attitudes reflected their belief that staff should be sympathetic to the aims and objectives of the Project. Their relative under-emphasis on caring skills reflected their feelings that the Division could provide care staff with the necessary skills during the training period and the view that "the majority of children with mental handicap are cared for at home by parents who acquire the necessary skills in the day-to-day situation".

The Objectives of the R.S.W. Training Programmes

Barnardo's in their application for funds to the D.H.S.S. in June 1981 stressed the importance of staff training and provided a "shopping list" of training topics. The senior personnel in the Division had to turn this shopping list of training needs into a coherent programme. They saw the training as a means of developing the right work practices, especially through the development of attitudes, and the development of group working as well as the development of child care skills. One tutor described the participative style of the programme in the following way:

> I don't think lecturing actually alters people very much. I think you have got to in fact get them involved in making their own decisions then they are far more committed. So, it was very

much from a workshop point of view... It is fortunate that the Project Leader took the view that the group should make a lot of the decisions themselves and take the responsibility.

Comment

The selection and training of staff were seen by the senior personnel of Barnardo's as two aspects of the same process. Senior personnel were concerned to ensure that the R.S.W.s had the right attitudes, and especially that they understood the principles of normalisation, that the R.S.W.s were willing and able to work together as a team and that R.S.W.s had the necessary skills to provide child-oriented care.

4.3 THE PROCESS OF THE SELECTION AND TRAINING OF RESIDENTIAL SOCIAL WORKERS

The Selection of R.S.W.s

The selection of R.S.W.s followed the conventional pattern of recruitment for residential units. The agency advertised the posts in local papers and specialist journals. People who enquired were sent a job description and a standard application form. After the closing date for the applications, a short-list was prepared and individuals were invited for interview. For each phase of the Project some 18 applicants were invited for interview for five R.S.W. posts.

For each phase there were two interview days and approximately half the short-listed applicants were seen on each day. The days were divided into three parts - a preliminary session, followed by "filter" interviews in the morning and formal interviews in the afternoon.

The Preliminary Session The day started with a general session for all the applicants. In this session divisional managers described the background to the Project and explained to the applicants the objectives and nature of the Project. In their talks they stressed the normalisation philosophy and the ways in which this philosophy would be used as a guide to child care. They also emphasised commitment - the commitment made by the agency to the children and the commitment required from the R.S.W.s.

The Filter Interview Following the introductory session each applicant was interviewed by one or two members of the interviewing panel. These were fairly short informal interviews designed to eliminate about three of the 9 applicants. Each interviewer had a standard list of questions. These were:

> What about the job appeals to you?
> Why do you want to work with children with profound mental handicap?
> What do you think you have to offer the project?
> You will be a very responsible member of the team and are therefore undertaking a very responsible job. What do you think the responsibilities might be?
> This is an unusual piece of work. In what ways is it different?

Following the morning interviews, the panel met to discuss the applicants. The first interview and the subsequent discussion were relaxed and informal. The interviewers were trying to exclude the weakest applicants at this stage and select only candidates who they felt should undergo the full rigour of a formal interview.

The Formal Interview After lunch all the interviewers joined one main interviewing panel. There was no set list of questions but each interview followed a similar pattern, the chairman introduced the panel and started with questions about the applicant's current post and previous experience, then interviewers dealt with different aspects of work in the Project and there was a concluding set of questions by the chairman about the applicant's attitude to different aspects of Barnardo's and its policy.

Following the interview, each applicant was discussed and each member of the panel gave the applicant a score out of five. In the discussion the panel attempted to assess the applicant's ability to care for the children, their sympathy with the approach of the Project and their ability to work with other R.S.W.s as a team. The discussion and decision-making were difficult because only two or three of the 6 applicants could be appointed. One discussion about a university graduate with experience of working with mentally handicapped people in a religious community illustrates some of the concerns of the panel:

> *Chairman* He is a sound caring person. I look favourably on him but he must be looked at in the light of the other

members. He has a high degree of intelligence. This could be very threatening. It could make the others feel very subdued and inadequate....He could be a powerful fellow.
Interviewer 1 He understands about relationships and menial tasks. He might overwhelm the others.
Interviewer 2 He coped well with the interview. He came out well. However, as an R.S.W. he might throw the balance out. The others wouldn't have his powers of perception or verbalisation. There were lots of traces of humanity. He would have to be told bluntly to live his life his own way.
Interviewer 3 I am bothered. He would cause an imbalance in the team. Nobody comes up to his level. It would be hard to put the brakes on him.
Interviewer 2 He's too far on for the others.

This applicant was not offered a post.

The formal interview was a difficult experience for both the interviewers and the applicants. Based on the application form, references and evidence from a 30 to 45 minute formal interview, the panel had to assess an applicant's suitability for work in the Project.

Applicants selected for social work posts There were 13 social work posts in the Project: one project leader, two A.P.L.s and 10 R.S.W. posts. The social workers selected for the Project were relatively young. The overwhelming majority of R.S.W.s were under 30 as was one of the A.P.L.s. One of the three senior workers and 7 of the 10 R.S.W.s were women. Most of the social workers had undertaken some post school education but only the Project leader had a professional social work qualification. Three of the social workers had been trained as nurses. Several R.S.W.s had pursued university degree courses. Six of the 13 had relevant qualifications; the Project leader had a certificate of qualification in social work, one A.P.L. was a General Registered Nurse, two of the R.S.W.s were State Enrolled Nurses on the Mental Subnormality Roll, one R.S.W. had a degree. The social workers' experiences of residential work varied widely. Six of the 13 had worked in a residential facility before, but none of the social workers had had extensive experience of residential work.

The selection of social workers was both important and difficult. There was no ready-made stock of experienced, qualified and skilled labour for the Division to draw on. Instead the Division had to attract applicants from a variety of backgrounds and, through a filtering process of short listing and

The Selection and Training of the Staff

interview, select the best individuals. Heavy reliance was placed on interviewing. As interviews tend to favour the articulate and self-confident, the interviewing panel were concerned to create a balanced team and to consider the personalities and skills of specific applicants in relationship to the whole Project and to other R.S.W.s. The interviewers selected a variety of individuals with a variety of backgrounds, education, qualifications and residential experience. Some of the R.S.W.s had previous experience of residential work with mentally handicapped people, others had very little experience.

The Training

In this section we shall describe the organisation of the programme of training for the second group of R.S.W.s. We shall discuss the training scheme in relationship to the overall objectives especially the development of child-care skills, the development of team spirit and the development of the right attitudes.

The Overall Programme The training programme had five weeks of mainly class-based sessions followed by 8 weeks of practical work with the children in the hospitals. The teaching in the first five weeks took place mainly in a room at Barnardo's divisional headquarters. The only exceptions to this were the visits to hospital to see and work with the children which started in the second week, the visits to the first and second set of bungalows in the fourth week and the shopping trips to Liverpool to buy items for the bungalows that were made in the fourth week.

Although there was overlap between the sessions, most sessions could be classified in one of five categories: development of child-care skills, team building, attitude development, provision of information and preparation for work in the hospitals. More sessions were devoted to the development of child-care skills than to any of the other objectives. Seventeen sessions were primarily concerned with the development of child-care skills in comparison to 13 sessions on team building, 10 sessions on attitude development, 7 on background information and 6 on preparing for work in the hospitals.

The sessions on *child-care skills* started in the first week with a description of the children and their needs. In the second week the R.S.W.s were introduced to the concept of an individual care plan. In the third week the R.S.W.s were provided with specific

The Selection and Training of the Staff

techniques for developing care plans. At the end of this third week, a day was devoted to the discussion of the link worker and to the selection of link workers for individual children. Before this session the discussion of child-care skills was fairly general. Individuals had not been given responsibilities for specific children. After the session the discussions were more focused as R.S.W.s now had specific responsibilities. The sessions on the specific development of child-care skills ended in the fourth week with sessions on goal-planning and reviews of practical needs. After this skills were developed through the work in the hospitals when the R.S.W.s worked with individual children on the hospital wards.

Child-care skills dominated the first three weeks of the programme and *team-building* dominated the second part of the programme. The R.S.W.s were asked to make key decisions, e.g. on the role of the link workers. Certain purchases for the Project, such as bedding, were left for the R.S.W.s to make. The emphasis on team building and participation gave the overall programme its distinctive style. Whereas the teaching of child-care skills was done by a range of teachers, the majority of the team building sessions were chaired by a polytechnic lecturer, who played an important role in facilitating group decision-making.

The third group of sessions was devoted to the *development of attitudes* amongst the staff working in the Project and especially in explaining the principles of normalisation and their implications. The key session on normalisation took place at the start of the second week. The bulk of the sessions on various aspects of the philosophy of the Project took place in the fourth and fifth weeks of the programme. A range of workshop leaders were involved in these attitude formation sessions.

The fourth objective of the training programme was to provide *information* about the operation of the Project and of the agency. This type of traditional teaching was kept to a minimum. There were information provision sessions at the start of the programme and again in the fifth week. The information provided at the start of the programme outlined essential background agency policies. The information in the fifth week of the programme concentrated on issues that had to be discussed but were not seen as central to the operation of the Project. Generally these issues were handled by the workshop leaders except the research component which was managed by the research team.

After five weeks, the R.S.W.s *started to work with the children in the hospitals*. This part of the programme underwent changes. In the initial planning stages this period was seen as a relatively short transition. The ward nurses were told by their managers that it would be three days and they felt that three days was not long enough. The course organisers decided to extend the period to two weeks for the first group of R.S.W.s. In the second phase the period of work was extended to 8 weeks and the R.S.W.s were prepared for this work by the assistant Project leader from Phase One.

Comment

Compared to traditional training programmes there was a relatively low emphasis on provision of information in a traditional classroom setting. As Barnardo's is a social work agency some basic information about agency practice had to be provided in this way but this was kept to a minimum. In contrast there was a high emphasis on the development of child-care skills, on team building and on the development of the right attitudes. The type of skills, the nature of the team and the attitudes emphasised were determined by the overall philosophy of the Project.

The model of work used by senior Barnardo's personnel provided framework for the training programmes. The senior personnel wanted to create residential social workers who were committed to normalisation, who were able to work together as a team and who put the interests of the children before their own personal interests. These objectives in turn shaped the overall structure and form of the training programme. Most of the sessions were designed to encourage active participation of the R.S.W.s either through discussion, through role play or through the allocation of specific jobs to groups of the R.S.W.s. The emphasis was on learning through participation.

4.4 ASSESSING THE SELECTION AND TRAINING

In this section we shall discuss the success of divisional managers in selecting and training staff for the Project. As we have already briefly discussed the sort of people selected for the Project in Section 3, we shall concentrate on divisional managers' perceptions of staff selection. We shall then discuss the training

The Selection and Training of the Staff

programme in terms of the divisional managers' and staff's perceptions.

The Selection of the Staff

Generally divisional managers felt that they had selected staff who could provide the right sort of care:

> I think we have a core of quite good people who were able to take on board some of the values, take on board that no matter how good we were, families were better. I think in the main we got a fairly solid group, evidenced by the fact that most stayed with us.

Divisional managers were less happy about the A.P.L. appointments. Whereas they felt they could provide R.S.W.s with the necessary care skills during the training programme, they felt it was more difficult to give A.P.L.s the necessary combination of management and care skills. Divisional managers acknowledged the problems they had in selecting and training people for A.P.L. posts but felt that these reflected general inadequacies in existing forms of training. The divisional managers were so concerned about the supply of suitable people for these posts that they developed their own divisional training programme.

The divisional managers had reservations about the process of staff selection. Social work agencies in general and Barnardo's in particular see formal interviews conducted by panels of managers as a key element in the process of selecting staff for residential units. The divisional managers had their reservations about panel interviews. They felt that these interviews could be misleading.

In the initial selection procedure, divisional managers had supplemented formal panel interviews with an introductory session and informal interviews. They developed this model by shortening the introductory session and replacing the informal interview with a discussion session with the Project staff, an observed leaderless group discussion and a written account of a cartoon about handicap. The discussions with Project staff were designed to help applicants get a more accurate feel for the Project and to give Project staff an input into the selection process. The visit to the Project was designed to provide the applicants with more information about the reality of working in the Croxteth Park Project. A divisional manager described the purpose of the observed leaderless discussion in the following way:

> They (the applicants) sit in a circle round the table and they are given a piece of paper with 14 questions or issues on it. Kind of things we might get are "we spent £220,000 on these houses for 8 kids would it have been better to use the money refurbishing a hospital ward for 20 kids?" ... We make notes about what people are saying, who are they talking to, would somebody fight a child's corner? If gives us a good picture of their attitudes to people with handicaps.

The last additional element in the revised selection process was a written commentary on a health education cartoon. At the end of the morning session each applicant was given a cartoon picture of a handicapped person meeting a dentist. The applicant's were asked to write a short account of the picture.

With these adjustments, divisional managers were happy that they had developed a selection procedure which would successfully identify applicants' basic attitudes and would enable them to select the right staff for the Project.

The Training Programme

We shall concentrate on the staff view of the training programme. We shall discuss the trainers' views first and then the R.S.W.s' views.

Tutors' Views The tutors generally felt that they had been successful in developing child care skills. None of the tutors identified any specific skills that they had overlooked. They felt that they had been successful in giving the R.S.W.s an interest in caring for the children. There were problems in developing this interest and commitment. In each programme there were periods in which the R.S.W.s displayed impatience and a desire to take on more responsibility. The tutors recognised this impatience and saw it as a positive sign of interest.

The second major objective of the programme was to develop group decision-making and the team spirit. One tutor was quite optimistic and felt that they had succeeded in building two integrated teams. Another was more sceptical and suggested that the only way of assessing this aspect of the scheme was to see how the R.S.W.s actually worked in the Project. He said that the R.S.W.s at the end of the training programme had gone through a process of the sharing and making decisions but their mutual understanding had not yet been tested in everyday work.

The tutors felt that the commitment of the R.S.W.s to the principle of normalisation varied. Some R.S.W.s had accepted and understood normalisation and incorporated it into daily practice whereas others still needed help in translating it into daily practice. The tutors said that they knew before the programme that there would be an important personal variable in the understanding and acceptance of normalisation.

The tutors attached considerable importance to the style of teaching. They wanted an integrated programme in which the different aspects of the programme reinforced each other rather than conflicted with each other and in which there was an integration between learning and doing, i.e. between explaining principles and applying those principles to caring for the children.

The importance of the integration of theory and practice led some of the tutors to emphasise the ways in which they drew upon the existing knowledge of the R.S.W.s and moulded this knowledge through various group processes. The tutors wanted the R.S.W.s to use the key concepts of normalisation to shape their practice. They wanted the R.S.W.s to discover the implications of these ideas, to understand their implications and to translate them into specific caring strategies. The tutors felt that they had not been able to fully explain this new approach to training to the R.S.W.s. They felt that the R.S.W.s still saw practice as doing things and still wanted to be taught specific skills.

Overall the tutors felt the induction programme had been successful. One tutor described it in the following way:

> I think, the very fact that an organisation will take on staff four to five weeks before a project gets off the ground and allows you to do this kind of initiative, I think that is great... This opportunity of starting a project and having the staff and being able to build up the thing from scratch rather than getting the building and everything and just get staff and tell them these are your rotas and this is how you are going to work. I would hope that this is a good step forward.

All the tutors thought the period of work in the hospital had been successful and had formed an essential link between the training programme and the work in the Project:

> I realise that it's sometimes not very pleasant being in there...
> But I think that when they come into the bungalows they will
> reap their rewards because they will know these children.

The tutors felt that the programme was a success and had achieved its objectives. The R.S.W.s were provided with child-centred skills, worked together as a team and understood the principles of normalisation. They felt that the programme was more successful with some R.S.W.s than with others, but these differences could be attributed more to personality factors than to the training. The tutors felt that the overall process of learning had been successful. The R.S.W.s had taken on the responsibility for decision-making. The criticisms made by the R.S.W.s were generally interpreted as signs of the success of the course, i.e. that they wanted to get to work with the children earlier and have more practical work.

R.S.W.s' Evaluation of the Training The trainees agreed with their tutors about the main objectives of the training programme. They defined it as finding out about normalisation, developing a team and learning about and caring for the children.

The R.S.W.s clearly understood the purpose of the sessions on normalisation and accepted the principles as set out in the sessions. Individual R.S.W.s differed in the extent to which they drew on these concepts and the sophistication with which they presented the ideas. Some R.S.W.s interpreted it as an anti-institutional philosophy. Others saw normalisation more in terms of normal life for the children and in developing the potential of the children. Generally the R.S.W.s accepted both the philosophy and the method of teaching and acknowledged the impact of the training programme on their own attitudes and perceptions.

There was, amongst the R.S.W.s, some disagreement about the development of teams. Some R.S.W.s felt that successful teams had emerged by the end of the programme. Some R.S.W.s felt, as did some of the tutors, that being a team in a training programme was far easier than being a team running the Project. The R.S.W.s identified the period of hospital experience as a special problem in developing the teams. During the hospital programme the R.S.W.s were in two separate hospitals and this created problems of cohesion and communication between the team.

The R.S.W.s accepted the child-centred approach of the tutors and they believed that the development of various child-centred skills was important. For example, the R.S.W.s accepted the reviews of the children as an important part of both the children's life in the Project and of their work with the children in the Project. They believed that the role play of a child review provided them with firm understanding of the structure of reviews and an insight into some of the tensions. However they felt that they had on occasions been taught these skills in a vacuum. For example, the sessions on the child profiles presented by the educational psychologist in the first week had stimulated a lively discussion on how to identify the needs of the children and how to develop care to meet these needs. Some R.S.W.s felt that they were unable to test out these ideas until much later.

The R.S.W.s did not accept the tutors' definitions of skills. They felt that in addition to skills such as goal planning they also needed specific nursing skills. For example, one of the children needed tube feeding. The tutors identified this need and one suggested that they should deal with the problem as it occurred in the Project. The other tutor suggested that the R.S.W.s might need to learn this skill and the R.S.W.s agreed with this second view. The R.S.W.s practiced tube feeding on each other so that they could not only learn the skill but also experience how it felt to be tube fed. They felt they needed skills not only to care for their children but also to establish their identity as competent carers in the eyes of people they would come into contact with such as the parents and the hospital staff. The R.S.W.s had special difficulties in this respect as these other individuals usually had a clearly defined status and competence. Parents could draw attention to their role as natural parents of the children and the nurses in the hospital could draw attention to their nursing qualifications. Most of the R.S.W.s did not have equivalent qualifications and yet needed to establish that they had the necessary knowledge to take over the care of the children.

The R.S.W.s all found participatory decision-making both difficult and emotionally demanding. The R.S.W.s appeared to accept its benefits but they did not like the costs, especially the length of time involved in coming to a decision. All of them found it difficult to adjust to this style of training as they had been used to more formal teaching. They felt that this style of training was productive but difficult.

The R.S.W.s identified a problem of relating the training programme to their work with the children. Some of the R.S.W.s felt that in the training period they were merely play acting and

The Selection and Training of the Staff

that no one was really tested out. Even having to make difficult decisions was seen as part of a game rather than as part of the real job of caring for the children. Indeed, some R.S.W.s suggested that success in these decisions could be misleading and might conceal real tensions and clashes of personality.

The work in the hospitals presented a different set of problems. In the hospitals the R.S.W.s had no formal status, they had to work with a range of different people and the objectives of the work were not as clearly defined. A major problem concerned the provision of information. There appeared to be some confusion about who was responsible for the collection and provision of information about the children. The R.S.W.s had started from the profiles of the children, prepared by the psychologists. These profiles were based on information collected by the educational psychologist from hospital staff and from psychological observations and assessment. The R.S.W.s appreciated the provision of this information but felt it did not provide a comprehensive picture of the children. They wanted to obtain more information about the children. However, when they first visited the hospital they were specifically told by the tutors not to interrogate the staff about the children.

There were also problems about the quality of the information. The tutors wanted the R.S.W.s to concentrate on developmental information about the children and on social information about their background. The R.S.W.s recognised the importance of this information but felt they needed more medical and nursing information. The R.S.W.s wanted to know the children's medical diagnoses and prognoses. They considered them important. They wanted this information because everybody else had it and because their status as carers for the children was somehow seen as related to this type of information.

The R.S.W.s saw the Project as a challenge to traditional services and felt they were scrutinized by the various professionals that they came into contact with. They needed all the knowledge that these professionals might have or use in addition to their own knowledge about normalisation and child care. The R.S.W.s felt that some of the information they received was inaccurate.

The R.S.W.s felt that the hospital staff saw them as competitors. R.S.W.s, especially in Phase One, felt that they did not receive adequate support from their tutors. The R.S.W.s felt that the hospitals had not been given a clear description of the Project and its objectives. They were forced to both explain the

The Selection and Training of the Staff

Project and even to defend themselves:

> I felt that our position (in the hospital) wasn't made clear. I think they (the tutors or senior Barnardo's personnel) should have gone into the hospital... I know they did go in and I'm not sure to what extent they did, but nobody seemed aware of what we were really doing... You know how stories get distorted. Nobody knew what we were trying to do.

The R.S.W.s felt that they did not get sufficient support from senior personnel of Barnardo's while they were in the hospital. Once a week the R.S.W.s in the hospitals met to exchange experiences with the group and with the tutors. At these meetings they presented their diaries of their daily work with the children. They did not feel that these sessions were properly used nor that their diaries were taken seriously. The R.S.W.s needed reassurance in a difficult situation and they felt that they did not get this.

Comment

As consumers of the training programme, the R.S.W.s were rather more critical than the tutors. Overall the R.S.W.s accepted the objectives of the training, appreciated the teaching methods used and felt that the period in hospital was both useful and interesting. In only one respect did the R.S.W.s challenge the overall conception of the programme. They felt that basic nursing skills and basic medical information had been underplayed and under-valued by the tutors. They felt that this information was not only useful in caring for the children but also important in establishing their status and credibility. In some respects these feelings must bring into question the extent to which the R.S.W.s accepted normalisation. They indicate that the R.S.W.s thought that the children had special needs that could only be managed with special skills. The R.S.W.s recognised this potential conflict but suggested that parents of children would also want this type of information and these types of skills and therefore it was normal for them as carers to seek this information and these skills.

4.5 SUMMARY AND COMMENT

The divisional managers saw the Project as a major service innovation and a challenge to the existing pattern of service. For this innovation to succeed they believed the Project had to avoid institutional practices which were implicit in some aspects of current training such as nurse training programmes. Senior personnel believed that it was important that the Project selected the right people and provided them with the right training.

The selection and training were seen as two parts of the same process. Selection was a screening or filtering process. Through this process the senior personnel of Barnardo's wanted to recruit a group of individuals who had the potential for running the Project in the right way. They did not want to recruit people who had traditional attitudes and were therefore cautious about employing qualified nurses. As a result the majority of the R.S.W.s did not have professional qualifications or extensive experience of caring for mentally handicapped children. The training programme was therefore extremely important to the success of the Project. In it, the tutors had to explain the principles of normalisation, and develop a team that could implement these principles through child-centred care.

The tutors rejected traditional classroom techniques. There was very little formal teaching in the programme. Instead the tutors constructed the training programme around various participatory teaching methods: group discussion, role play and group decision-making. The tutors saw their role as helping and guiding the group to reach certain decisions and acquire certain attitudes.

The tutors were generally happy with the programme. They felt that they had managed to give the R.S.W.s the necessary work skills, they felt that the R.S.W.s could act together as a team and that they undertook the principles of normalisation. They did have reservations about specific R.S.W.s but these were seen as inevitable consequences of different personalities rather than evidence of the failure or shortcomings of the training programme.

However, the R.S.W.s had criticisms of the programme. Some of them found it difficult to adapt to the needs of participatory learning. Many had had little previous experience of role play or group decision-making and felt that they needed more guidance in this area. Some felt that major topics had been neglected.

The Selection and Training of the Staff

There was a general concern that medical information and nursing skills were undervalued in the training programme. These were seen as essential not only in identifying the needs of the children and providing care but also in establishing and maintaining the status of the R.S.W.s as competent carers. The R.S.W.s found the learning style both difficult and demanding. There were criticisms of the period of experience in hospitals. The R.S.W.s felt that the tutors were not clear about the purpose of the hospital experience and had not adequately prepared the hospital staff for their work and had not provided adequate support for them while they were in hospital. However the R.S.W.s did believe it was an essential part of their training and really did prepare them for work with the children.

Overall the R.S.W.s thought the programme was a success. They recognised and accepted the objectives of the programme. They liked the participatory style of training and they felt that the period of experience in the hospital was both useful and essential.

5 THE SELECTION, PURCHASE AND CONVERSION OF THE BUNGALOWS

BIE NIO ONG AND ANDY ALASZEWSKI

We start this chapter with a discussion of the importance of selecting the right buildings for community-based units. We then describe and evaluate the way in which the Division selected, purchased and converted the four bungalows that constitute the Croxteth Park Project.

5.1 HOUSING FOR RESIDENTIAL CARE

Reformers and philanthropists at the beginning of the 19th century were concerned that the majority of dependent people were neglected and that few were housed in appropriate accommodation. The move to improve treatment was associated with a move to design and build special types of accommodation. The legacy of the 19th century was a network of purpose-built facilities or institutions (Alaszewski, 1986).

Since the Second World War, researchers and policy-makers have questioned both the scale and nature of institutional provision (Jones and Fowles, 1984). Although the criticism of institutions has been generally accepted, the search for a generally accepted alternative has proved difficult, especially for people whose behaviour is so challenging or health problems are so great that they could not live independently in the community.

In the 1950s and 1960s, agencies with the responsibility of providing an alternative residential service purchased and converted large old houses or built residential units. The choice was usually pragmatic and depended on a variety of local factors including the local housing stock, the local land market, the availability of capital grants and the specific client group.

In the 1970s a more explicit theory of care has developed to justify and guide choice: normalisation. An important aspect of normalisation is providing a suitable physical environment in which individuals can develop their own personalities and skills. O'Brien and Tyne have contrasted the dehumanising characteristics of the traditional institution with the individualised environments required for normalisation. They argued that the physical environment could and should provide opportunities for personal choice and for the expression of individuality and personality. They argued that this would occur when

> * Arrangements encourage self-expression in furniture choice and in the selection and display of decorations. There is adequate space for people to use or display at least some personal furniture and decorations, and there is adequate storage space for other possessions and furnishings.
> * Space arrangements not only permit privacy but also give a clear sense of "personal space". Staff do not intrude on personal space without invitation or permission.
> * All facilities are accessible to people with physical disabilities.
> * There are active efforts to make spaces, especially living spaces, not just physically comfortable but pleasing and even beautiful. (O'Brien and Tyne, 1981, p.13)

Not only should the physical setting of care allow for individual choice and expression, it should also allow the individual to interact effectively with his or her social environment. To achieve this the setting should have the following characteristics:

> * The service is situated in a place which makes it easy for people to get to and use a wide variety of valued resources.
> * The programme is located so that it is easy for a person to maintain contact with his/her family and home community.
> * There are imaginative efforts to give people access to valued places.
> * Services are kept numerically small and do not themselves congregate so many people as to make it impractical for those served to make frequent use of community resources. (O'Brien and Tyne,1981, p.22)

The Jay Committee (1979) was heavily influenced by the normalisation philosophy. The Committee was specific about the type of physical environment in which it expected residential care to be provided. The Committee felt that units established in ordinary houses would create the preconditions for individualised care, in which staff respected the individuality of each person and encouraged each person to develop to his or her maximum potential. The residential unit would do this by creating a range of normal experiences from which mentally handicapped people could learn.

The Use of Ordinary Houses for Residential Units The D.H.S.S. has created a number of special initiatives to move long-stay residents out of hospital. One of these initiatives is the Care in the Community scheme. Twenty-eight pilot projects have been funded by the D.H.S.S. Some of the projects make use of purpose-built accommodation either because of the specific needs of the clients or because suitable properties are not available on the private market, but most use existing houses (P.S.S.R.U., 1985, p.3).

In the report of a conference on moving mentally handicapped children out of hospital, Shearer described four schemes that provided alternative patterns of residential care for mentally handicapped children, in Skelmersdale, Ashington, Winchester and Camden. All made use of existing houses that had been converted. In his foreword, Sir George Young, Parliamentary Under Secretary of State at the D.H.S.S., commended this development in the following way:

> I must give just one example: the ordinary terrace house in Ashington, Northumbria, which now provides a real home for children from Northgate Hospital. As Julie's mother said, "it's the smell of baking that greets you when you go in, instead of the smell of disinfectant that hits you on the hospital ward". (Shearer, 1981, p.3)

Although there is a trend towards establishing residential units in ordinary houses, there are few published accounts of this process. One exception is the work of Wessex Health Care Evaluation Team. Wessex was the first Regional Health Authority to adopt a consistent policy of moving mentally handicapped people out of institutions and into small units in the community. They started at the beginning of the 1970s with small (20-25 place) purpose-built units sited in the community and designed to provide services for mentally handicapped people living in a specific catchment area (Felce et al., 1984, p.170; and Mansell et al., n.d.).

As the programme developed in the 1970s, so its objectives were refined with increased emphasis on the quality of care provided for mentally handicapped people in the community and the use of the normalisation philosophy. The research team responsible for monitoring and encouraging the changes encouraged experiments with the establishment of residential units in ordinary houses. The first house was opened in November 1981, the second in April 1983 and several more are planned. The concerns with normalisation were very clear in various aspects of the selection and conversion of the first house. The planning team selected an ordinary house that was close to local amenities and avoided external alterations that would distinguish the house from others in the neighbourhood (Felce et al., 1984, pp. 170-1). The house was furnished as far as possible with materials and equipment found in an ordinary house rather than in an institution. Internally the house was adapted to provide a normal living environment and attention was paid to implementing one of the main themes of the normalisation philosophy - an age-appropriate environment:

> Decoration and furnishing is to a standard that would be expected in our own homes and care is given to choosing fittings, equipment and personal materials which are appropriate to people's chronological as opposed to mental ages. (Felce et al., 1984, p. 171)

As in other community units there was a tension between the desire to create a home-like atmosphere and the need to satisfy various regulations for residential units. The house did have to have some fire-safety features that would not have been found in a normal house (Felce et al., 1984, p.171), but efforts were made to minimise the obtrusiveness of these features (Mansell et al., n.d., p.1).

The D.H.S.S. Works Group has published two pamphlets (1981a and 1981b) that evaluated existing residential units for mentally handicapped people in the community and provided guidance for subsequent development of these units. The Works Group felt that the physical environment had an important influence on the nature of care received by mentally handicapped people (D.H.S.S., 1981a, p.10). The Works Group surveyed a number of developments by health authorities, personal social services departments and voluntary agencies. The group clearly favoured units that blended into the local environment and that were like ordinary houses. For example, Barnardo's Lineside Close Unit was criticized because "administrative offices and residential accommodation for staff are on the same site creating a large complex" (D.H.S.S., 1981a, p.20). On the other hand, the Works Group commended the way in which the houses of the Barnardo's Skelmersdale Unit blended in with the other houses and "none of the houses can be identified as any different from others on the estate" (D.H.S.S., 1981a, p.20).

The Group was influenced by the ideals of normalisation. For example in their evaluation of residential units they stressed the importance of not differentiating the units from their environment:

> The arrangement of buildings within a site can diminish or enhance their similarity to "ordinary" housing ... The more buildings resemble local housing the more favourably they are accepted by the neighbourhood. Unusual external appearances ... can make the buildings noteworthy as being different rather than achieving the aim of blending in with the surrounding buildings and may suggest that the people living in them are unusual in some way. Thus some of the destigmatising potential of community-based facilities can be lost (D.H.S.S., 1981b, p.39).

A similar concern with creating a normal environment can be found in the Work Group's discussion of the internal organisation of residential units (D.H.S.S., 1981b, p. 39).

Comment

The move away from institutional care to care in the community was initially shaped by criticisms of existing services. There was in the 1960s no clearly defined alternative and local agencies responded pragmatically to the local land and housing situation.

In the 1970s the concepts of normalisation began to filter into England and Wales. The normalisation philosophy stressed that mentally handicapped people should be treated as highly valued members of society and that they had the right to enjoy the same experiences as other citizens. If mentally handicapped people needed residential facilities then these should allow easy access to and integration in the community and should create an environment that was appropriate to the age of the residents and which allowed for their personal development.

This model of residential care has influenced the plans of several health and social services agencies. A series of experimental projects have been established in ordinary houses. In all these schemes great attention has been paid to ensuring easy access to community facilities, to ensuring the unit cannot be clearly identified as a residential unit and to ensuring a home-like environment.

5.2 THE OBJECTIVES OF THE DIVISION FOR THE SELECTION AND CONVERSION OF THE HOUSES

Key members of their working party, the Divisional Director and the Barnardo's architect, had both visited community programmes in the U.S. The architect described the influence of his visit in the following way:

> I had been to the States to look at the housing developments for this type of child and studied the potential implications and it was very useful to see what was considered to be impossible over here actually in practice there... (We started from the position) that these children can and have a right to live in houses.

The main objective was clear, the Project had to use normal housing so that the children could experience normal living. However, the working party wanted to find houses that were considered desirable and attractive by other people. The Divisional Director stated his view in the following way:

> We are going to care for the most problematic of children in this field, in an ordinary setting and, through moving them into an even better setting, we enhance them. Doing it in a nice place, in a posh estate reflects well on the kids.

In the application to the D.H.S.S., Barnardo's stressed the importance of acquiring accommodation in the right sort of area. The area had to constitute a well-balanced neighbourhood and have a range of community facilities that could be used by the unit. The houses should have

* a quiet domestic situation, typical of the immediate neighbourhood;
* a likely supply of potential volunteers preferably within walking distance. It follows that small isolated housing areas will not be suitable;
* a closeness to shops, parks, public transport and schools;
* an absence of steep slopes, steps or changes of level that would provide exceptional problems for wheelchair-bound persons and
* (a neighbourhood with) a variety of "ages" of residents and social groups. (Barnardo's, 1981c, pp.10-11)

The neighbourhood should avoid some of the negative features that were typical of many areas in Liverpool, including

* vandalism and exceptional social problems (including isolation in high-income areas);
* dangerous roads, airport noise and industrial nuisances. (Barnardo's, 1981c, p. 10-11)

In line with the normalisation philosophy Barnardo's felt it was important that the buildings selected did not identify the Project as special residential accommodation. It was important that the buildings used should blend in with other buildings in the neighbourhood. As many of the children would have physical handicaps, Barnardo's wanted ground floor accommodation with a sunny garden.

Internally the buildings were to resemble a normal home and allow the children to develop their own spaces. Barnardo's did plan to adapt the buildings to the special needs of the children. However they were also clear that these alterations should be "child-centred" and should only be made in response to the specific needs of specific children:

> The building must adjust to the children's needs where possible, and unlike a hospital, the limits of these alterations will be the same as for their parents' homes and for the community based accommodation it is hoped they will grow into as adults. Personal possessions and school work should take pride of place and the building must accommodate these. (Barnardo's, 1981c, pp.11-12)

Barnardo's envisaged making alterations for two other reasons: to minimise disruptions to neighbours and for fire precautions. The fire precautions potentially involved important modifications and Barnardo's accepted that these had to be incorporated.

The Division did not see the Project as a long-term facility. It was hoped that a substantial number of children admitted to the Project would move into other care settings, especially into family care. Although the houses had to be suitable for the care of profoundly handicapped children, it was also important that they could be adjusted to the needs of different children. The Division did not subscribe to the view of the working party establishing community units in Portsmouth and South East Hampshire health authority that

> In our experience, it is better to identify the family group of young people first, and then go "home-hunting" based on their individual needs. (Abbott and Chamberlain, 1986, p.50)

The Project was not a long-term facility and therefore had to be flexible enough to adjust to the needs of different children.

Comment

The senior managers in the Division were heavily influenced by the normalisation philosophy. The buildings had to signal to the community that Barnardo's believed that the children were highly valued members of society. Therefore cheap and second-rate accommodation was unacceptable. Barnardo's wanted accommodation that was desirable and highly valued.

Barnardo's developed a series of fairly specific criteria for the location and nature of the buildings. The buildings had to be located in desirable areas. They had to be located in areas with suitable amenities, such as shops, parks and schools. The buildings themselves had to avoid the stigma of institutions, either by association, e.g. being located near institutions, or through appearance. Internally the buildings had to be home-like and child-centred. Although alterations would have to be made to the buildings in the interest of the children these alterations should not destroy their home-like character.

5.3 THE PROCESS OF SELECTING AND ADAPTING THE HOUSES

Selecting Houses on Croxteth Park Estate

Although the Division were committed to using ordinary houses, the Division had to decide what sort of houses they were going to use and how they were going to obtain them. In terms of the buildings, there was a choice between using two-storey houses, bungalows or flats. Most families, who own their own house, live in a two-storey house, therefore there was likely to be a reasonable supply of these properties and they would be seen as normal family houses. On the other hand these houses have staircases, which create problems for disabled people. Bungalows are more suitable for disabled people but there is usually a short supply of bungalows and they have a relatively high market price. Flats are often suitable for disabled people, especially if they are on the ground floor. There is a relatively short supply of flats for purchase as most have been constructed and are owned by local authorities or housing associations.

The working party decided that accommodation should be on the ground floor, either in a flat or a bungalow, as two-storey houses could not be readily adapted. The architect was the main advocate of purchasing flats. He argued that, as the Project was an experimental demonstration unit it was important to show the children could live and be cared for in flats as well as houses. The architect did not have much support within the working party. Other members of the party felt there would be practical problems in using flats and the working party decided to look for bungalows.

Barnardo's could have obtained the properties it required by renting from the local authority or housing association or by buying on the open market. As the Division had used rented housing for a project in Skelmersdale, senior managers felt they wanted to do something different. The decision to buy bungalows was influenced by the housing stock in Liverpool. Liverpool is a city in decline. Most metropolitan areas are deprived but Liverpool is especially deprived. The inner city council estates have been described as having "a proportion of vulnerable and low skilled groups unparalleled in Britain outside Glasgow" (Liverpool Area Health Authority, 1979, p.8). This deprivation

The Bungalows

results in mutually reinforcing health and social problems. The housing problems of Liverpool considerably limited the available accommodation even outside the deprived areas. Much of the housing outside the inner city was being developed specifically to rehouse people from the inner city.

The Division decided to buy on the open market but the type of property purchased depended on the availability of funds. As part of their application to the D.H.S.S. Barnardo's specifically requested funds to purchase and convert the properties. The D.H.S.S. made a £100,000 grant towards the initial cost of the scheme.

Once the D.H.S.S. had made this decision, the architect and building inspector began to look seriously for the right properties. In the north-east part of the city they found a new housing development, Croxteth Park. Broseleys, a national company, had purchased two large areas of land and planned to build a large community with a variety of houses and a range of facilities including shops and a community centre.

Buying houses on the estate had several advantages. Barnardo's could buy pairs of bungalows and could make alterations to them before they were built. The Project would be part of the community from the start. The architect felt that this was an important factor:

> If you try and buy houses in established middle class communities you've got to build up a relationship with the neighbours before you do anything like try and find the premises. In the time it takes to get planning permission and with the neighbours round the premises, the premises have gone off the market... Croxteth Park looked to be a development over 7 or 8 years of a very large community. Croxteth itself is a very troublesome run-down area with tremendous social problems. This looked to be a development in the countryside on the fringe of these social problems but there was sufficient amount of housing, schools and shopping development to start up a whole new community. We would be in ... right from the beginning.

The working party felt that the houses were desirable properties that ordinary families wanted to lived in.

Adapting the Houses

The main concern of the working party was that the adaptations should not alter the external appearance of the houses and therefore mark them out as a "children's home" and that the adaptations should not affect the resale value of the house. Externally the working party discussed two modifications, altering the layout to the drive at one pair of bungalows and building covered walkways between each pair of bungalows.

The initiative for the alterations to the driveways at Phase One came from the builders. The bungalows are set above the level of the road and getting wheelchairs to the houses would be quite difficult as the drives were quite steep. The builders altered this incline but the architect felt their alterations differentiated the houses from others and he redesigned the work.

Initially the architect proposed and the working group agreed to one other external change to the houses. They agreed to build a covered walkway between each pair of bungalows so that night staff could more easily supervise the children in each bungalow. When the plans were discussed at Barnardo's headquarters it was felt that these alterations would clearly differentiate the bungalows from other houses on the estate. The working party decided to abandon the walkways. The architect described this decision in the following way:

> The team (i.e. working party) all thought that they (the bungalows) should be linked. We went in the wrong direction. It became an institution, we were actually designing a small institution in the community and it wasn't until it was formally submitted, the whole package had been submitted to our head office that somebody jumped up and said "This is a small institution in the community. You have got so engrossed in the design that you have missed the basic philosophical point of providing small houses." So we scrapped all that and we said well we can cut out the link, take the risk and if we find a need for it we can build it later. It has turned out fine. All we did was put two doors into the sides of the houses so you could walk between the premises easily.

Although it is a general policy of Broseley's not to make structural alterations to the houses, they agreed to make minor alterations to the interior of the houses for Barnardo's. In all the

The Bungalows

bungalows the corridors were widened by 6 inches by redesigning the layout of internal walls. This reduced the "living space" but improved access for wheelchairs especially from the living room to the bathroom and bedrooms. The doors were also widened by four inches for the same reasons. There were relatively substantial alterations in the bathrooms. The bathrooms were increased in size and the baths placed on raised plinths to cater for the special needs of the children and to help staff.

As far as possible Barnardo's used the normal fixtures and fitments for the bungalows but repositioned some of them so that they would be more accessible to disabled children. The architect found it difficult to plan some of these changes as they had to be made before the selection of the children was finalised. The only major changes to the fixtures and fitments were the radiators for the central heating. The architect felt that as some of the children might be ambulant, ordinary radiators might be dangerous. Therefore he asked Broseley's to install low surface temperature radiators. These were large and rather obtrusive.

Generally Barnardo's found the builders very helpful and the building inspector felt they had tried to accommodate Barnardo's more than they would other clients. For example, they allowed Barnardo's to start work on minor alterations in the house before the contracts for the sale of the houses were completed. Similarly Broseley's had been quick to mend any defect. When Barnardo's bought the houses they received a two-year warranty and a six-month defect liability. The building inspector had heard from other residents that the builders were slow and sometimes reluctant to repair defects but Barnardo's experienced no difficulty. If there were minor defects, then the staff in the house contacted the site manager and he usually arranged for the repair work. If there was a list of minor problems or a major problem then the builders usually took rather longer and the building inspector had to contact the builders.

The final stage in the preparation of the house was the decoration, and the fitting of the carpets and the furniture. This was the responsibility of Barnardo's. Again the choice of these items was heavily influenced by the normalisation philosophy. They had to be age appropriate and suitable for the needs of each child.

One particular concern was that each house should have a different character. While the houses should in general look like other houses on the estate, each house had its own individual atmosphere with different furniture, carpets, wallpaper and paint. The building inspector, who joined Barnardo's when these decisions were being finalised, confessed that he found it took him some time to understand the full implications of the normalisation philosophy.

> I found it (the normalisation philosophy) difficult to understand as I was new to Barnardo's. I felt that with the normalisation philosophy there is a lot of attention paid to details, for example the wallpaper could be the same (in different houses) but it had to be put on different walls or they wanted to have different bells on each house.

The decisions about these items were made differently in each phase. In the first phase, the decisions had to be made before the appointment of the R.S.W.s. The domestic advisor from Barnardo's head office in London selected the decor and the major items of furniture. The process tended to be rather time consuming as all the decisions had to be approved in London. The R.S.W.s in this phase only selected minor items such as lamps, bedding and bedroom fitments. In the second phase the R.S.W.s were appointed before the completion of construction and therefore they were involved in making all these decisions.

The Impact of Regulations

The Project is a residential home and could be registered as a home under the Registered Homes Act. Registration confers certain advantages, particularly on adult residents, e.g. they can claim various social security allowances, but it also has disadvantages. The home must be inspected and approved by the local authority. Generally agencies establishing community units in ordinary houses have found the alterations required by local authorities extremely intrusive, especially with the installation of smoke detection and fire fighting equipment and fire resistant doors. These alterations conflict with the objectives of creating a normal family home for the residents (see P.S.S.R.U., 1985, p.3 and Social Services Committee, 1985, paras. 132 and 134). In the application to the D.H.S.S., Barnardo's did not envisage making substantial alterations to the structure of the house but they did envisage making modifications to the internal structure to ensure that it was fire proof. Following internal discussions the Division

The Bungalows

decided to follow the principles of normalisation and only install equipment that would be found in other houses on the estate. There were no smoke or heat detectors and there were no fire-resisting, self-closing doors. Each bungalow had a small fire extinguisher and a fire blanket in the kitchen. The main precaution against fire was the careful instruction of all staff in procedures and a monthly fire drill. The Division followed the D.H.S.S. suggestion of adopting a policy of sensible compromise (D.H.S.S., 1985, para. 23).

A similar problem existed with registration under the Registered Homes Act. The P.S.S.R.U. noted that the regulations tend to impose an "institutional standard on domestic properties" (P.S.S.R.U., 1985, p.3). The Barnardo's architect discussed the initial plans with the local authority and they raised no objection. But since then the new Residential Care Home Regulations have been issued as part of the Registered Homes Act. These regulations might involve substantial changes in both the structure and activities in the Project and would run counter to the principles of normalisation. For example notices about hygiene etc. would have to be displayed, the washing machines would have to be moved out of the kitchen. The Division discussed registration with the Liverpool City Council. The Council's view was that Barnardo's did not have to register the Project as a Home as there were only two children in each house. The Division decided not to register. However they accepted the spirit of the Act and felt that there should be quality control of residential facilities, therefore they invited the local authority to inspect the Project as if they were registering.

Comment

Drawing on experience of services in the U.S., the Barnardo's working group felt it was important that the Project should be established in and make use of ordinary buildings. There was a wide choice of the sort of buildings that could be used, and the ways in which these could be obtained. The final decision to purchase bungalows on Croxteth Park Estate was dictated by a desire to balance the requirements of the normalisation philosophy for ordinary housing that was generally considered desirable, with the special needs of profoundly and multiply handicapped children and with the availability of property in Liverpool. The conversion and equipping of the houses was dominated by the concern to ensure the bungalows looked like ordinary family houses and did not stand out as a residential unit.

5.4 ASSESSING THE USE OF ORDINARY HOUSES

The Location of the Project

Advocates of normalisation argue that residential care should enhance the social status and image of mentally handicapped people. Barnardo's did this by buying desirable properties. They adapted them so well it was difficult to distinguish them from other homes on the estate. However, buying new houses on a new estate had costs.

There was limited public transport on the estate and the second pair of bungalows were quite a long way from the bus stop. At night the walk from the houses along deserted roads could be quite intimidating. This tended to act as a barrier to people who did not have their own transport, involved the Project in quite high transport costs and created parking problems.

In line with the normalisation philosophy no special arrangements were made for car parking. The first pair of bungalows were in a cul-de-sac. There was only space for three cars in front of the houses. Staff parked their cars in the drives which led to the garages but these were relatively short. There were occasions when the drives were full and there were quite a lot of cars parked along the street. The parking at the second pair of bungalows was rather better. The drives were the same but there was more on-street parking as this pair of bungalows was situated near a T-junction. There were occasional parking problems when a large number of people had to come to the Project, for example for a child's review. Parking has not caused any tension with the neighbours.

Since one of the objectives in selecting houses for the Project was to locate them in an area with easy access to such community facilities as shops, general practitioners, schools and leisure facilities, we examined access to these facilities. The Transport and Road Research Laboratory of the Department of Transport has developed measures of accessibility. Some of these measures were extremely sophisticated (for a review of these accessibility measures, see Jones, 1981). As these measures tended to be surveys of accessibility to specified facilities for various social groups (e.g. Jones, 1984, Joint Working Group, 1981 and Pickup, 1984) rather than case studies of the access from specific households they were of limited use for our study. They do draw attention to some important aspects of accessibility and the effects of spatial location and mode of transport (Mitchell and Town, 1977, p.2).

The National Travel Survey for 1972/73 indicated that three main forms of travel, car, bus and walking, accounted for 94% of all trips (Mitchell and Town, 1977, p.3):

> Trips (for) education and shopping are much shorter than are those (for) the other two major trip purposes (work and social visits)... Education and shopping trips are more commonly made on foot... This suggests that these facilities are more often available locally... Education and shopping trips are also more likely to be made by children or women, who both have a low probability of having the use of a car. (Mitchell and Town, 1977, p.3)

In terms of the personal characteristics of the traveller and in particular their ability to use a car, Mitchell and Town argued that with the growth of car ownership from 0.05 cars per person in 1951 to 0.25 cars per person in 1975 and with a likely ownership of 0.45 cars per person by the end of the century, two distinct groups of travellers have emerged, those with the use of a car and those without (Mitchell and Town, 1977, p.2).

Like other residents on Croxteth Park, the staff and children in the Project were very much part of a car-using culture. As part of the education of the children, they were taken on various forms of transport including buses, trains, the Mersey Ferry and even donkeys, but for routine travel, public transport was impractical. A bus ride needed two staff for each child.

We examined accessibility in terms of access on foot or by car to shops, health facilities, schools and leisure facilities. As the estate was new and had few community facilities, apart from a General Practitioners' Surgery, which was established on the estate in 1985, most of the facilities were some distance from the Project and were only accessible by car. For example the nearest "corner shop" selling groceries was 30 minutes on foot from Phase Two and the school attended by most of the children was over 20 minutes by car. Although reports from other residential units indicate that they also rely heavily on cars for the travel needs of severely handicapped residents, most appear to be located nearer to public transport and community facilities (see for example the Fareham Unit, Abbott and Chamberlain, 1986, p.50).

The lack of public transport did not affect the children's mobility, as they would not use it routinely. It did however make the Project relatively inaccessible for people who did not live locally and who did not have the use of a car. In particular volunteers, without their own transport, found it difficult to get to the bungalows. As most volunteers tended to visit the Project in the evenings, they found the walk from the bungalows to the bus stop along deserted roads intimidating.

The Internal Structure of the Project

Each house had its own individual atmosphere with different furniture, decorations, pictures on the wall and photographs of the children. For example, one house had a bird cage whereas another house had a cat. At birthdays and Christmas the houses were decorated in the same way as other houses on the estate.

In some ways space was used in the houses in the same way as in other households. There was a living room that was used for leisure activities such as listening to music and entertaining guests. The dining room was connected to the living room. The children sat at a table for their meals. They also used the dining area for some leisure activities such as painting. The kitchen was separated from the dining area by a door and was used for the preparation of food. All meals were prepared in the kitchen. The bedrooms were relatively small and could not be used as play areas. The children were always cleaned and changed in the privacy of their own bedroom with the door closed. At night they had a quiet period with one of the care staff, reading a story in their room or having a chat and a cuddle. The bathrooms had toilet facilities which were used by everyone. All the children's bathing equipment was kept in the bathroom and it also had other features that one would find in a normal bathroom such as a linen basket for dirty clothes.

However, these areas were also used for other activities that did not normally take place in an household. The living room was used for physiotherapy sessions as it had more space than any other room. It was also used for staff meetings and for general administrative activities. The kitchen tended to double as an informal staff room. One of the spare bedrooms in each pair of

The Bungalows

bungalows was used as a sleeping-in room and also provided a storage area where old notes, supplies and staff coats and personal belongings were kept. It also contained a notice board where staff communications were pinned up. The other spare bedroom in each pair of bungalows was used as an office and had a telephone.

The bungalows were relatively small and space had to be used efficiently. Living space was always given priority and determined the characteristics of the bungalows. For example, meetings and administration took place when the children were not at home. There was a problem of storage. Like many modern houses storage space was minimal. The lofts and garages were used to store equipment but a lot of play equipment had to be put behind sofas in the living room or put in cupboards. The only problem in moving around the house was carrying children between their bedrooms and the bathroom. Children were undressed in their own room and carried to the bathroom. With older heavier children this could be quite a strain for the staff and following discussions storage units were placed in the bathrooms and the children could be changed on these.

Children from the neighbourhood often visited in the afternoon and the living rooms were then turned into play rooms. These sort of visits were welcomed and the atmosphere was one of an ordinary house where friends drop in. When official visitors came to look at the Project there was pressure on space. The Project Leader tried to limit visits to times when the children were at school. But it was inevitable that sometimes a child would be off sick and the visitors had to be received in the living room whilst a child was carrying on with his or her own activities. The number of visitors was restricted when the staff felt that they were becoming too intrusive.

The children in the Project had birthday parties and these were organised in either the living room or, weather permitting, in the garden. All these parties were successful and at some over 15 children came as guests. There was sufficient space to play games such as "pass the parcel" and to dance and these occasions have contributed greatly to the quality of life of the children and to their relationships with the neighbours.

The use of the gardens was relatively limited. Although they all had play equipment, there was no direct access to the gardens from the houses. All the bedrooms were at the back of the house between the main living areas and the gardens. Therefore if the staff want to take the children into the garden on a warm day they had to carry chairs and other equipment into the garden. The gardens were not fully "established" and only had young trees and plants. This meant there was no shade and the children could not stay in the garden without protection from the sun. The staff were buying more equipment and furniture for the gardens so that they could be used more.

Comment

Advocates of normalisation stress the importance of enhancing the social status of people with a mental handicap. One way of doing this is buying and equipping houses to the highest possible standard. Barnardo's pursued this policy and the houses they purchased were undoubtedly very desirable. However, buying houses on new estates did have costs. There were limited community facilities on the estate and limited public transport. This could be a barrier to people who did not have their own transport and could involve the Project in quite high transport costs. The houses are small and have limited space and therefore the internal environment has to be carefully managed.

5.5 CONCLUSION

One of the first decisions the Division had to make when establishing the Project was about the type and location of property. Although the working party had a general idea of the sort of children that would be cared for in the Project, they did not have detailed information. Their choice of buildings was guided by the principle of normalisation and the availability of housing in Liverpool.

A major concern of the Division was that the houses should demonstrate the children were highly valued. They did not want second-rate accommodation. They wanted houses that ordinary families would like to live in. These houses had to be in a suitable location and be suitable for caring for the children. The Division identified areas in which they did not want to locate the unit. These included areas which had high rates of social problems, and areas considered undesirable because of traffic or industrial development. The Division also defined suitable locations positively in terms of easy access to community facilities.

The Bungalows

The objectives for the selection of the houses were defined very much in terms of normalisation. The Division wanted to use ordinary houses that could be used for the care of the children with a minimum of adaptation. In particular they did not want the houses to be different from other houses. They wanted to demonstrate that profoundly handicapped children could be cared for in ordinary houses in ordinary residential areas.

These general objectives had to be turned into more detailed guidelines so that the architect and building inspector could locate suitable premises. Barnardo's could have either rented or bought property. At an early stage the Division decided to buy rather than to rent. Buying gave the agency greater control and choice. The Division decided to buy bungalows as they were ordinary family houses that could be easily adapted to the needs of children with physical handicaps.

Identifying suitable bungalows was a difficult and time-consuming process. Following a year of searching, in which the architect and building inspector visited most of the new developments in Liverpool, they identified a new estate in the north-west corner of Liverpool. The houses on the estate were generally considered desirable, they were being bought by ordinary families and there was a range of housing, including pairs of bungalows.

The Division identified and purchased two pairs of bungalows at opposite ends of the estate and decided to make minimal alterations to the houses. The builders were very co-operative in adapting these bungalows to Barnardo's requirements. For example they realigned the drives on one pair of bungalows and they expanded the size of the hallways, bathrooms and doorways in both pairs of bungalows. Externally it is difficult to differentiate the bungalows from the houses on the estate, and internally there are a limited number of features that are distinctive, e.g. the radiators and the baths.

Buying new houses on a new estate did have its disadvantages. There were few facilities on the estate and travelling was expensive both in time and money. The houses were small and space had to be managed very carefully in them. However Barnardo's did buy and adapt houses that were generally considered to be attractive. Each house was distinctive and each house was a home and there were no features that distinguished them as institutions. They were attractive houses that indicated the value Barnardo's attached to the children.

6 PROVIDING CHILD CARE

ANDY ALASZEWSKI, GERRY DODSON AND BIE NIO ONG

The central activity of any residential facility is the provision of care for the residents. In the first section we discuss general issues of child care. We then examine Barnardo's objectives for child care, the processes they used to achieve these objectives and assess the extent to which they achieved these objectives.

6.1 STRUCTURING STAFF/CHILD RELATIONS

Within social services, residential care is a branch of social work. Care staff in children's homes are often referred to as residential social workers. Although field work is usually seen as the major source of professional development, there is growing awareness that models of practice developed in fieldwork cannot be directly transposed into the residential setting and residential care requires its own models (see, for example, Walton and Elliott, 1980). The two forms of social work share similar objectives, e.g. improving clients' skills and abilities so that they can perform their social roles competently, but they operate in very different contexts and use very different strategies. Most field social work is based on the casework model with its intermittent one-to-one relationship between client and social worker in a private setting, e.g. the client's home. Residential social work is based on a continuous relationship that often involves a group of clients and a group of social workers and interactions usually take place in a more open setting, i.e. the residential unit.

In the field social work setting the relationship between social worker and client is usually structured through a case-allocation system. A client is allocated to a social worker who then takes responsibility for the case. When the interaction is short-term and limited to the profession this form of management can be effective. However, when the interaction is longer term and involves other professionals then an additional problem of co-ordination develops. In this situation, a key-worker system may be used, i.e. one professional takes overall responsibility for the case, takes the lead in planning the client's therapy and acts as a link between the client and the other professionals. The key worker model has also been used in residential settings. For example, a joint working party of the British Association of Social Work and Residential Care Association (1976) saw the key worker as either a field worker or residential worker. The key worker would be responsible for planning and implementing an individual's care plan and would be accountable in the agency for the case.

The Barclay Committee on the role of social workers clearly saw the key worker as an important feature of good practice in residential social work. It argued that the model was appropriate for all clients in residential care, but particularly children and young people, as they

> are at particular risk of finding that responsibility for their lives and problems is divided between a number of people - e.g. a field social worker for links with the family, a residential worker for life in the home and no one in particular for forseeing and planning what is to happen after departure. It is our view that one agreed and appropriate person should concern himself with, and accept formal responsibility for, the client's needs as a whole. We give unqualified support to the concept of the *key worker*. (Barclay Committee, 1982, p.69)

The Barclay Committee saw the key worker as a planner and co-ordinator of services. In addition the Committee, implicitly drawing on the psychoanalytic theories of child development, identified a second key relationship for each child - a parenting relationship.

> For satisfactory emotional growth and development every child needs, we think, the unconditional commitment of at least one person (usually mother or father, or both). For a child in residential care this person may be someone outside a residential establishment or foster home. Sometimes he or she will be found only within the residential setting. Each child in long-term care needs such a person and one of the

> tasks of the key worker is to make sure, whenever possible, that a committed adult is available to the child. (Barclay Committee, 1982, p.70)

The Wagner Committee felt that key workers could provide continuity of care:

> The continuity which comes from having consistent attention from staff whom an individual can come to know well and trust, is an important aspect that has to be planned, managed and coordinated. This is one reason why the development of residential "key workers" as a means of establishing some continuity of care should be encouraged. (Wagner Committee, 1988, p.63)

Both the Court Committee (1976) and the Warnock Committee (1978) identified the fragmented and disorganised nature of services as a major shortcoming in the services for children with a handicap. The Warnock Committee felt these shortcomings could be overcome through a key worker or named person system. The different agencies and professionals in contact with a family and a child should agree that one professional would act as the main contact for the family and child:

> One person should be designated as Named Person to provide a point of contact for the parents of every child who has been discovered to have a disability or who is showing signs of special needs or problems. (Warnock Committee, 1978, para. 5.13)

The All-Wales Working Party on services for people with a mental handicap also identified the key worker as the linchpin of the new pattern of services in Wales. The working party described the role of the key worker in the following way:

> A named person should be assigned as the main point of contact with each mentally handicapped person and family. The key worker may come from one of a range of disciplines... What is crucial is that the client and family have ready access to the expertise of the Community Mental Handicap Team and its contacts. This access will be most effectively provided if a key worker is identified as the main point of contact. (Welsh Office, 1983, pp. 24 and 28)

In field work, the key worker's main role is as a co-ordinator. In residential care, the key worker has an additional role. The key worker is usually in daily contact with the client. Thus an important aspect of the key worker's role is designing and implementing therapeutic programmes. These are often referred to as individual programme plans.

The starting point of comprehensive child care should be the individual needs of the child. Carle (1981) saw individual programme plans as a natural corollary of the view that people are unique and should receive the assistance appropriate to their particular needs in their specific environments. An individual programme plan is a statement of a child's needs and agreed activities for providing for these needs. All the participants involved in a child's care meet periodically to assess the needs of a child, to discuss the child's progress and to review the best way of achieving these objectives. The Jay Committee (1979, para. 93) saw review meetings as an important forum in which individual programme plans or "life plans" could be agreed. They argued that these meetings should involve both parents and professionals and that all participants should share in the decision-making. The programme would include a statement of long and short-term goals, the steps required to reach these goals, the resources required, the responsibilities of different participants and the mechanisms for reviewing and monitoring progress.

The development of individual programme planning was a central feature of the All-Wales Strategy. The Welsh Working Party recommended that services should be based on

> A system of individual plans (which) will help ensure that a team of relevant professionals is assembled around each client at regular intervals to agree objectives, to contact, to provide services and to review progress. (Welsh Office, 1983, p.28)

The working party specified that these plans should be based on regular six-monthly review meetings.

Comment

In residential care a team of social workers take responsibility for planning and providing the care of a group of clients. The way in which this care relationship is structured and monitored is central to the provision of care. Although the theory and practice of residential social work is not as well developed as field social work, it is clear that in most progressive settings, some form of key worker system is being used and these key workers have a crucial role to play in formulating and implementing individual programme plans.

6.2 CHILD CARE IN THE CROXTETH PARK PROJECT

In the original application to the D.H.S.S., the divisional managers placed Barnardo's and the Croxteth Park Project in the mainstream of child care practice when they stated that

> Residential care is not an end in itself...the majority of children in Barnardo's residential care are placed for more sustained periods with the objective of enhancing their capacity either to return to their own families long-term or to prepare for living with a substitute family or to achieve a greater degree of independence and fulfilment in less dependent forms of "sheltered" or residential care. (Barnardo's, 1981c, p.2)

The Croxteth Park Project was placed within this overall philosophy. The division planned to take children with a profound mental handicap and provide them with the necessary care and support so that they could move onto family or other suitable placements. The Project was to enhance the children's development and prepare them for alternative placements. To achieve this divisional managers emphasised the importance of providing each child with an individual programme.

Programme planning was to form an essential part of the process of preparing the children for alternative placements:

> This project intends to demonstrate...that appropriate individual development programmes, devised by a multi-disciplinary team, can bring about improvements in the condition of the children, and a reduction in their levels of dependency so that when they leave the ISU they may remain in the community... The whole working environment, ethos and pattern of staffing will be conducive to those therapeutic ends (i.e. of the plan). (Barnardo's, 1981c, p.4)

An essential part of the process of care was to be the

relationship that each child developed with adults in the project.

> The aim will be to ensure as far as possible that each child always has one adult offering him exclusive attention ... The child/adult contact will not be haphazard, but will be consciously planned as part of a curriculum developed individually for each child. (Barnardo's, 1981c, p.4)

In the original application the discussion of adult/child relations was relatively generalised. As the planning of the Project developed, so the role of different members of staff was more clearly specified and in particular 8 of the 10 R.S.W.s were defined as link workers. The link worker was not only to be the child's key worker but was also expected to act as a substitute parent. The divisional managers wanted link workers to develop an emotional bond or attachment with their child (Bowlby, 1965 and Fahlberg, 1979). The Project leader described the development of this role in the following way:

> From the inception of the Project, staff were involved in defining the roles they were to play. They called the role in relationship to the children in their care "link worker" who in essence was asked to be willing to "love" his/her link child. The link worker has to understand that the nature of this love means showing warmth and affection, means protection and defending, means representing and advocating.

The development of the link-worker role was a conscious rejection of some of the traditions of professional practice, in particular the tradition that care staff should maintain a degree of detachment from their clients. The divisional managers wanted to use the emotional attachment that developed between link worker and child as part of the therapeutic process. The Project leader described the therapeutic role of this attachment in the following way:

> The children coming to our service had, as a result of living in long-stay institutions, experienced few opportunities to build up close relations with significant adults... They had come to equate physical and verbal contact with care tasks such as feeding and dressing, and had little experience of close and loving interaction for its own sake... We viewed emotional investment of staff in a child as beneficial for a child's personal growth and ability to develop social interaction. We

asked workers to "contractually" engage themselves in a committed relationship with the child and take on the responsibilities of a surrogate parent.

The attachment was a means of preparing a child for family placement. The divisional managers felt that once children had developed an attachment to one adult, they would find it easier to learn to attach to another adult. The link worker had to accept that although they would, for a time, be the most important person in a child's life, other adults could and should take over this position. The Project leader described this aspect of the link worker's role in the following way:

> The growth and development of the child as the result of this relationship (with his or her link worker) was not an end in itself, but was considered to be a step towards building a future with meaningful relationships. This means concretely that the link workers were working towards rehabilitating the children with their natural families, finding foster families for them or other suitable community provision. As a logical consequence of the application of the normalisation philosophy ... family life was considered a desirable goal and staff had to learn to cope with transferring the emotional relationship to families.

Comment

As a child care agency, Barnardo's is in the forefront of developments in child care. In developing a model of child care for the Project, the Division drew on current thinking about the role of residential facilities in child care. A major concern was that placement in the Project was not an end in itself but part of the child's overall development and in particular a way of moving children out of long-stay hospitals and into more suitable placements in the community such as foster families.

6.3 MANAGING STAFF/CHILDREN RELATIONSHIPS

In this section, we shall discuss the processes through which divisional managers structured staff/children relationships. We shall consider the formal processes used to structure and monitor these relations and we shall examine the role of the link workers.

Therapeutic Planning

Review Meetings As a child-care agency, Barnardo's had a statutory duty to undertake periodic reviews of all the children in its care. The Division had adopted a policy that children in residential projects should have six-monthly review meetings to assess their progress and to plan their future. In the Croxteth Park Project, a major function of the review meetings was developing and monitoring the implementation of each child's individual programme or therapeutic plan. The overall purpose of the meetings was to set medium- and long-term objectives for each child and to identify the methods through which these objectives could be obtained.

The membership of the reviews reflected their function. To achieve effective planning it was important that the meeting provided a forum in which all the people involved in a child's care could pool their information about the child's development, could contribute to a discussion about areas of potential development and could agree a plan of action for the next six months. Thus while Barnardo's staff took the lead in initiating the meeting and formed the core of the meeting, they also issued invitations to all individuals who had a significant part to play in the child's future. This included the children's parents, teachers from the schools and, in some circumstances, volunteers.

The structure of the meetings was also related to their function. The meetings were held in one of the Project bungalows. To indicate the importance which the Division attached to the meeting, it was chaired by a senior divisional manager, usually the Assistant Divisional Director. The child's link worker played a key role in the review meeting. He or she set the scene for the meeting by describing the child's progress since the last review and identifying the major concerns of the Project care staff. Generally the link worker's report formed the "agenda" for the review and other members of the review tended to contribute to the discussion. Towards the end of the meeting the chairperson would summarise the discussion and identify areas in which the participants agreed. After the meeting the chairperson prepared a report that summarised the discussion and listed the recommendations of the meeting. This report was circulated to all the participants at the meeting and to all individuals concerned in the child's care. In the Project it formed the basis of the child's therapeutic programme.

Goal Planning The recommendations of the review meeting provided the general objectives for child care. The care staff developed a process of goal planning to convert these general objectives into specific short-term goals that could then be used as the basis for the day-to-day care of the children.

When the Project was set up, the Division's educational psychologist agreed to provide the care staff with advice on the children's developmental needs and on ways these needs could be met. The psychologist suggested that the care staff should adopt a goal planning mechanism through which they identified the specific skills they wished to develop and specific therapy programmes for enhancing these skills. The planning was to be a cyclical process of planning, implementation, and evaluation. During the training period the psychologist and care staff developed initial plans for each child. When the care staff started work with the children, they used the care plans as the basis of the children's daily care. The care staff maintained activity charts for each child which specified activities that should be carried out on a daily and weekly basis.

Initially the plans were maintained and regularly reviewed. However, in spring 1984, the educational psychologist went on maternity leave. This seriously affected the goal planning process. The care staff did not have confidence in their own abilities to develop and implement plans without specialist advice and support. There was little discussion of the plans and by August 1984 goal planning had become a ritual. There was very little alteration in specified goals and activities.

In August 1984 the Project leader accepted there was a problem with goal planning and consulted a psychologist. As a result of his discussions he decided to purchase a goal planning package which had been developed in the Wessex Region, the Bereweeke package. This arrived in September 1984. All the care staff and the Project leader were trained in the system. The Project leader took overall responsibility for the administration of the system. The two co-ordinator R.S.W.s took responsibility for writing individual programmes. The link workers were responsible for the implementation of the programmes.

Each child was assessed using the Bereweeke check list and for each child the staff identified an overall goal with specific weekly targets. These targets were based on a number of factors

Providing Child Care

including the children's skills and preferred activities, the staff's preferred activities with the children and the feasibility of the targets. The programme writers drew up charts with specific instructions about the type of activities which care staff should undertake and the times at which these activities should be undertaken. The programme writers were responsible for assessing each child's weekly progress and for adjusting the programme accordingly.

Communication

Although the Croxteth Park Project was small and all the participants knew each other, the staff accepted that good communication was essential for effective child care. There were two specific processes of maintaining good communications - record keeping and meetings.

Records The care staff accepted that good records were essential for effective child care. The children had a profound mental handicap and were therefore unable to speak and provide information about their care. Records were essential for maintaining continuity of care and treatment, for monitoring the children's progress and for identifying any emerging problems. Divisional managers saw records as more than just a method of ensuring continuity of care and monitoring the standard of care. They felt that the children had a right to a history. As the children could often not remember or record what had happened, the records could act as their history.

There was a continuous debate in the Project about the content and format of records. The agency had a clear policy that certain types of information should be recorded such as the children's medication and diets. However the precise format was not specified. Both phases of the Project developed a comprehensive child-centred system. In Phase One the staff had developed a range of specific records, e.g. diet sheets, sheets to record specific areas of activities and used a daily diary to record impressions or assessment about a specific child. In Phase Two most of the information was concentrated in each child's daily diary which had specific headings such as diet, mood, bowel actions, and individual needs (see Table 6.1).

Table 6.1
Types of Records in the Unit

Phase 1	Phase 2
Activity Chart	Activity Chart
Daily Diary	Daily Diary (including
Night Reports	diet, bowels etc.)
Diet Sheets	Night Reports
Bowel Charts	Specific charts for children
Specific charts for children	e.g. Ivan, clamping
e.g. David, catheter	Medical
e.g. Barbara, clamping	Goal-planning (Bereweeke)
Medication	Weekly Summary
Goal-planning (Bereweeke)	I Can-Do Book
I Can-Do Book Life	Life Story Book
Life Story Book	Home-School Diary
Home-School Diary	

Group Meetings The review meetings were a formal part of the establishment of the overall strategy of care. There were no equivalent regular meetings for goal planning. However each phase of the Project held a weekly group meeting. In these meetings, the care staff discussed operational issues such as staff rotas but they also gave presentations about the individual children. In both phases, the first item on the agenda was the children and their progress. For example on the 12th October 1984 a group meeting in Phase One discussed the progress of the three children they cared for and a fourth child who had been accepted for admission to the phase. One of the children, Linda, had just been admitted to the hospital for investigation of an eye complaint and the group heard about her progress.

The review meetings established the long-term plans for each child's care, and the goal plans formed the framework for the day-to-day care. The six-monthly review was a mechanism for all the people involved in a child's care to meet, to pool their information and to plan the child's future. The agreed plan was then circulated in a report. The goal planning mechanism had a similar structure. The goal plan represented an agreed set of short- and medium-term goals and prescribed activities. Information relevant to the plan was kept in each child's records and the group meetings were a way of pooling information about each child.

The Link Worker

The link worker role evolved during the training period preceding the opening of the first two bungalows in July 1983. The trainers provided the R.S.W.s with an outline of the ways in which they expected the Project to work. They suggested that each child should become the major responsibility of one of the R.S.W.s who should act as a "surrogate parent" and prepare the child for family placement. The Divisional Director told the staff:

> No matter how good Croxteth Park is, and we expect it to be very good, you can do better. We can place these children with families.

During the training programme, the trainers and the R.S.W.s discussed the ways in which the surrogate parent role should be developed. The discussions tended to focus on the problem of reconciling professional detachment with emotional commitment. The staff were concerned about becoming over-involved and over-committed to the children. However, as the R.S.W.s moved into the second part of the preparatory work and started work with the children in hospital so a structural method of reconciling emotional involvement with professional objectivity developed. Four of the five R.S.W.s became link workers and they were expected to develop a personal commitment to and emotional bonds with individual children. The fifth RSW was called the co-ordinator and together with the assistant project leader took on the role of maintaining an overview and ensuring professional objectivity.

The staff group selected the term 'link worker' because it had multiple meanings. It not only referred to the emotional attachment or bond but it also referred to the link worker's role as a bridge. This dual role was crucial. The staff recognised that giving each child the opportunity to attach to an adult provided valuable experience for the child. However if the attachment became too strong it might prove an impediment. The link worker might not want to share his or her child with other adults and in particular might try to block the child's progress to a foster family. The staff accepted although they could provide their children with

Providing Child Care

high-quality care, foster parents could provide them with even better care. Thus they were the child's link to other significant adults, particularly natural and foster parents. The bond between the link worker and his or her child had to be a bridge into family life.

The development of an emotional bond is a complex process, however, choice seems to be one aspect. Choice is usually seen as unprofessional. However in the initial selection of roles, the staff group accepted the importance of choice. They tried to match R.S.W.s to children according to the relative interests of the staff and the ways in which different children reacted to different staff.

Once this allocation had been made, the link workers started working with the children in the hospitals. They observed the ward staff care procedures and talked to the nurses about the children and their care. They worked alongside the nurses and gradually took over the responsibility for their child's care. While the staff were in the hospitals it was clear that the bonding process had started to develop. The children began to respond to their link workers and the link workers in turn started to act as advocates for their children. In this initial phase this led to tensions on the ward as some of the nurses felt threatened by the developing link and tended to see the link workers as over-enthusiastic and optimistic. In these circumstances the Project leader had to ensure that working relations were maintained.

When the children moved to the bungalows, the link workers could take full responsibility and could begin to use the emotional bond to enhance their child's development and to plan for their child's future. The bond formed the framework within which the more task-oriented work, such as goal planning and basic care, could take place. The link workers' investment in their child was high because they were responsible for and could take pride in their child's progress, behaviour and appearance. One link worker described the role in the following way:

> In the day-to-day life of the child the link worker has the dual task of being on the one hand a surrogate parent with all the responsibilities that that entails, and on the other hand the more difficult tasks of attempting to place himself in the child's shoes and making all the demands that in other circumstances the child would quite rightly be making for himself... The link worker has to be courageous and resilient, pig headed and determined - after all the quality of life of his link child is at stake.

The staff group organised a rota system so that the link workers could have as much contact with their children as possible. As the link workers did not work 24 hours a day, there had to be mechanisms for ensuring that other staff implemented the link workers' plans. Occasionally tensions arose when a link worker did not feel that the other staff were implementing the plans properly. These tensions were resolved through mechanisms such as group meetings. Individual link workers attached so much importance to the continuity of care that they often worked unpaid overtime to accompany their child to a hospital visit or visit the school.

To assist the link workers in developing bonds with their child, the Project leader arranged for a child-care specialist to act as a consultant and to help the link workers. Two link workers used the consultant to develop programmes which focused on nurturing and physical contact. For example, both link workers developed an individually tailored bedtime routine in which they cradled and stroked their child to create an atmosphere of warmth and intimacy.

One of the link workers' key roles was to prepare the children for fostering. The Division had established a fostering project in 1979 and a social worker from the fostering team was attached to the Project to help the link workers, to provide social work support for the families of the potential foster children and to work with the prospective foster families. The social worker from the fostering project saw the link worker as a crucial person in the fostering process. The link worker was a major source of information and could provide an informed view of the extent to which the child was ready for family placement. Once the decision had been made to place a child, then the link worker's role began to change. During the initial stages of the process the link workers played a dominant role. They were seen as the experts. They provided the foster parents with information and advice and they advised on the speed at which the relationship should develop. Once the relationship was established then the link workers developed a more supportive role. For example, they were involved in the provision of respite care. Five of the six link workers whose children had moved on maintained contact with their child and continued to provide support.

Comment

It was clear that all the children admitted to the Croxteth Park Project had been severely emotionally damaged by their experiences in hospital. Divisional managers wanted to repair this damage and prepare the children for placements in families. They wanted to create a caring environment that would achieve these objectives. The divisional managers accepted the views of the writers such as Bowlby and Fahlberg that the development of a relationship with a significant adult played an essential role in the development of a child. Therefore the link worker was given a central role in child care. Individual care staff were encouraged to develop close emotional relationships with the children and, through the medium of review meetings and goal planning, the relationship was exploited to provide the child with development opportunities and prepare the child for placement in a family.

6.4 ASSESSING THE IMPACT OF THE PLANNING PROCESS AND THE LINK WORKER

In this section we shall consider the process of care from the point of view of the children, the managers and the care staff.

The Children

In Chapter 10, we provide a more detailed account of the children's development. In this section we shall make some brief preliminary comments. There can be no doubt that both the overall planning and the goal planning were extremely successful. The Project successfully placed in foster care 6 of the original 8 children and in all cases the transition took place without undue stress for the children or the adults involved. The goal planning appeared to have been a similar success. The staff were able to devise and implement programmes that significantly improved the children's skills.

However there was one criticism. In the original model of care, short-term objectives, such as enhancing and developing the children's skills, were linked to the longer-term objective of family placement. Although the children's skills developed, there was no evidence that this was a crucial factor in the placement of the children. For example, the child, who in many respects has made the greatest progress since his placement in the Project, was not placed in foster care. Relationships with natural parents were the crucial factor in the fostering process. Children, whose parents either had little contact or did not object to family placement, were placed. Children, who had a significant relationship with their parents and whose parents wanted them to stay in Croxteth Park, stayed.

Divisional Managers

Generally the divisional managers felt that the process of child care had been very successful. They felt that the children had developed emotional bonds with their link workers and these bonds had been positively exploited. Children had developed emotionally, socially and intellectually and had moved on to foster care.

The divisional managers accepted that there had been problems initially in the goal-planning process. The initial system had been heavily dependent on the support of professional staff, especially the psychologist, who helped design it. When this psychologist had no longer been able to provide support, the care staff did not have sufficient confidence in their ability to develop new goals. However the divisional managers felt that the Bereweeke system resolved many of these problems. They did need the support of a psychologist to establish the system but once it was operational, its clear structure and allocation of roles and responsibilities meant that it required little external support.

The divisional managers were very pleased with the development of the link worker system. They felt that all the link workers had developed an intimate relationship with their child and this relationship was based on love and respect. The link workers were committed to their children and acted as advocates.

The divisional managers did recognise the dangers of emotional involvement. The high levels of commitment meant that staff were often working long unsociable hours. During periods of staff shortages, there was a danger that some staff were becoming physically and emotionally exhausted. The managers accepted that staff would, on occasion, feel under stress but felt that this stress was very different from the burnout exhaustion, which has been identified in many residential facilities (Cherniss, 1980 and Pines, 1983). Burnout is a form of emotional and physical exhaustion that results in staff leaving the facility. The divisional managers felt that the exhaustion, which staff felt on occasion in the Croxteth Park Project, was more like the exhaustion experienced by parents, i.e. tiredness, feelings of guilt and frustration when goals were not achieved. The divisional managers felt that care staff could cope with these feelings if they were given adequate support. We shall discuss the nature of this support in the next chapter.

The divisional managers recognised that the system had serious costs for managers, particularly in terms of staff flexibility. Staff were not interchangeable. It required a high level of staffing to maintain the link worker system. Thus managers were faced with a dilemma. Although the Croxteth Park Project had generous staffing levels, when compared to other residential projects in the Division, the staff in the Project often complained about the low level of staffing.

Establishing and maintaining the link worker/child relationship over a long period of time was difficult. In the short term staff sickness or leave were difficult to cope with and in the longer term there were problems when staff or children left. The Project leader considered different methods of dealing with this problem. One possible solution was to have a more family-like model, i.e. two link workers caring for two children. The divisional managers felt that this would create too many management problems and would diffuse personal responsibility for care. They did, as a temporary expediency, agree to a job sharing scheme. Two R.S.W.s, who were on secondment to a training course shared their link worker role with two part-time R.S.W.s. The managers felt that this arrangement led to increased problems of communication as the joint link workers were rarely on duty together. However they did not feel that the children suffered. Indeed the children seemed to enjoy having two relationships.

As the Project developed, so a new problem began to develop. Initially Barnardo's had specified that the children admitted to the Project should not only have profound mental handicap but they should also be young. They wanted time to work with the children. Thus most of the children initially admitted were under 12. But as the Project developed so the children tended to get older. This was partly the product of the natural ageing process; the children who were not considered for fostering were getting older. It was also a product of the changing demographic structure of the hospital population of children. As the hospital authorities were moving the younger children out first, so the remaining children were older. As a result several of the residents in the Project were no longer children, they were young adults. The divisional managers felt it was important to adjust the caring process of this change. To do this they drew on the normalisation philosophy and considered the changing relationship of young adults to their families. As children grow into young adults so their close ties with their parents loosen and they begin to develop relationships outside the home, often with other young adults. Their home usually remains a significant place but they tend to treat it as a base.

The divisional managers felt that the young adults in the Croxteth Park Project could make a similar transfer. Their experience of attachment to a significant adult had given the opportunity to "fill" the emotional and development gaps caused by their institutional past. For some of these young adults Croxteth Park would become a home for life. For these young adults, the link workers could provide a bridge to a supportive social network and to a locality. The Project could act as a base from which they could develop a range of activities and relationships.

The Care Staff

The attitudes and views of care staff about working in the Project and providing care tended to fluctuate. When they first started work, the care staff were full of enthusiasm and commitment. In many respects they had been "charged up" by the training programme and convinced of their ability to provide a higher standard of care than the hospitals. However as they began to get a more realistic picture of the amount of work involved and the level of resources so the staff experienced a sense of anti-climax. This reached something of a crisis point in March 1984. During the winter of 1983/4 the sickness rate had risen amongst both staff and children. In the last week of March 1984 two of the children were in hospital, two R.S.W.s were ill, two R.S.W.s were on leave and one post was vacant. Only five of the 10 R.S.W.s were available for work. During the week, all the staff available had to work extra hours.

During this crisis period all the care staff told us that they were still committed to their children and to the overall concept of the Project. However they were critical of the support they received. Some R.S.W.s even told us that they felt they were being exploited. The Project had promised a lot and demanded a lot of commitment and made them feel guilty if they did not provide the required level of commitment but they felt that they received little in exchange. Although these R.S.W.s did develop a more positive view of managers when the crisis passed it did show that staff often felt under heavy stress and required a lot of support.

Some staff expressed reservations about the impact of the system on the development of relationships between children and members of staff, other than the link workers. Sometimes the latter could become too involved with their own child to the detriment of the Project as a whole; they might show less interest in other children, or exclude others from involving themselves with their link child. Furthermore, link workers found it difficult to accept opinions or constructive criticism from other staff because "they know what is best for the child". All these inherent difficulties had to be addressed either in group meetings or in supervision.

Despite the reservations about some aspects of the link worker role, most of the link workers felt this way of working gave them great job satisfaction and that they positively gained from the experience. Since the link worker experience was so personal, we shall conclude this section with one link worker's account of her relationship with her child.

> It is difficult to know where to begin - the beginning you might say - but where that beginning is is hard to say. Was it way back in September 1983 when I first met a mischievous brown-eyed little boy showing off by knocking bricks down, or was it eight months further on in time when after much deliberation I took him on board as my link-child?
>
> My argument at the time for becoming Rob's link-worker was that I knew him, having worked within the Project and surely this was better than introducing someone new into his life again. I can see myself now - sitting in the Office at Crucian Way "spouting" all my so-called justifications - the challenge of a new child with his potential - the relationship that we already had - a chance to utilise more of my teaching skill and training. Notice how at this stage none of them were actually very "Rob" orientated. They all sound very good on paper but in reality they all came way behind what Rob and I actually gained from our time together. "Magic" is the word at this stage that I choose to describe our relationship.
>
> In the initial stages my perception of the link worker role

was based on theory and my own experience as a parent. The problem lay, however, in the fact that I saw only what I could give to Rob and what he could gain from our so-called contact - drawn up mainly by me and other members of staff. I chose Rob - not he me. I often wonder if at the time he would have chosen differently. It did not take me long however to realise that he was just as capable of giving as receiving and that our relationship of link worker and link-child was definitely a two-way process.

And so it was that I enthusiastically commenced my role very methodically or so I thought... I wrote a complete new file for Rob, stating aims and objectives just as I would have done with a class of children in previous years. How naive I was and how tolerant Rob was of all the new things I was eager to try with him, but most of the time I remember him being highly amused at my "antics". It was as if he knew that in time I would realise what I really had to offer him.

He did not particularly want sophisticated goal plans, he could have these any time and from anyone. He wanted me to love him and to care for him just as any Mum would for her child. It was though, in a sense that he knew he was entitled to this. It was at this point, about two months into our "contract" that I knew I was "hooked". Gone were the official aims etc. and goal plans. Life for Rob as far as I was concerned was going to give him all he deserved, mainly the knowledge that somebody cared for and loved him for himself, not just because he was a physically handicapped child.

The real work then began, just as any Mum would fight for the rights of her child, I began to do so for Rob. I made my presence known within the Project, within the school and in later days, within the Organisation, in order to get Rob what he needed - a family. Again on paper this sounds all well and good. In reality it meant that each day that passed was a day nearer the time I would inevitably have to give him up.

Our time together was a lovely mixture of "the good and the bad". He will never know the guilt I felt at having to go off duty, going on leave and finally giving him up. I argued with staff as to how he should be treated, I resented the fact that we were an institution. Why should he have to live like that? One problem that I lost sleep over, quite literally was when he frequently woke up crying in the night. Night staff and day staff alike theorised over an approach to the problem. All I saw was a little boy waking up in the night desperate for some security. Yes I knew all the problems - "He could make a habit of it" etc., but I never ignored my own children, I gave them what they needed, a cuddle and the knowledge that I was always there.

Rob never spoke to me as such, he communicated through facial expressions. As I write this I can see him now expressing all the emotions a five year old realises: curiosity, fear, insecurity, joy, love, pleasure, pain, distaste.

He could make me understand some of his innermost thoughts just as I hope he understood mine. If I was tired or down he would in his own way comfort me. If I was displeased with him, he would either get very upset or more often than not do his utmost to make me laugh and get round me.

Throughout our relationship I had nothing but positive expectations for Rob but the closer I got to him the more I related to the feelings I think I would have encountered as his natural parent. "Why was Rob the way he was". I vividly remember one day seeing a young Mum out with a baby in a pram and a young child about the same age as Rob walking beside her. I was resentful that Rob was in a wheelchair and not walking like this young child. I bottled up a lot of resentment at this stage.

When the time finally came for Rob and I to part, I was split down the middle, half of me wanted what I had always wanted for him, a family, the other half initially could not stand the thought of anyone else taking over my role. Much support, encouragement and understanding helped me through this and the realisation that I could not commit twelve months of my life to someone and forget them overnight.

I had previously thought that I would be fine in a few weeks. Those weeks stretched to months during which I battled with resentment, jealousy and the pain of loss. On the surface all was well and to most that enquired I was "coping well" with the situation, very naturally so, that is what I had fought for was it not?

It is now four months since I finally placed Rob in the care of his foster family. I shall miss him. Most of all I miss the privacy I once shared with him, but what I miss is overshadowed by what I see now. Rob taking his place in a family where he belongs!"

6.5 SUMMARY AND COMMENT

The central activity of a residential project is providing care for the residents. This care is predominantly provided by the care staff and therefore the relationship between care staff and the children is vitally important. In traditional facilities care staff were often provided with little positive guidance on the ways in which to develop relations. In the Croxteth Park Project, the managers drew on progressive elements of social work practice to provide care staff with positive guidance on the ways they should interact with the children. The link workers were asked to develop close emotional bonds with their children. This relationship was exploited for positive therapeutic benefits. The long-term objectives were established in the review process and were concerned with such issues as the child's best placement. Short-term goals were established through the goal planning process. There can be no doubt that the processes were successful in both enhancing the children's development and in enabling the children to move into foster families. However, the relationship between these short- and long-term objectives was not clear. The model of work adopted was highly demanding for both care staff and managers. Link workers had to make a high commitment to the Project and the children. In exchange for a high commitment they tended to experience a high level of satisfaction. Managers had to ensure that link workers had the necessary resources and support.

7 STAFF MANAGEMENT AND SUPPORT

ANDY ALASZEWSKI, BIE NIO ONG AND HEATHER ROUGHTON

In this chapter we shall consider the ways in which divisional managers managed and supported staff. In the first section we examine the issues involved in staff management and support in residential care. We then examine the type of management and support which divisional managers wanted to develop in the Project.

7.1 STAFF MANAGEMENT AND SUPPORT IN RESIDENTIAL CARE

In welfare states, welfare agencies profess to serve the interest of their clients. Despite the public commitment of policy-makers and service managers to this principle, the reality can be very different. Many clients do not see these agencies as acting in their interest. They perceive welfare agencies, as at the best unhelpful and at the worst as hostile (McKinlay, 1975, p.366). Although senior managers in these agencies may espouse progressive client-oriented policies, they do not, in practice, have much contact with clients. They delegate the provision of services to front-line workers who often have very different values and attitudes. The activities of these front-line workers are difficult to observe and control (see, for example, Lipsky's discussion of street-level bureaucrats, 1980).

Within institutions, the power and autonomy of front-line workers has been a major impediment to reform. Belknap (1956) in his study of a state mental hospital in the U.S., found two separate value systems. The official value system was professionally-based and was based on publicly stated aims of treating and rehabilitating patients. However the dominant value system was based on attitudes of front-line workers that patients could not be treated or rehabilitated but at best could be trained to provide cheap labour to reduce the costs of running the institution.

In social work, the management of front-line staff has been a particular concern. The clients of social work agencies are often poor or vulnerable and social workers have considerable power to alter the lives of these clients. Supervision is one method of ensuring that front-line workers do, indeed, implement agency policy. Parsloe (1981) defined the tasks of the supervisor as:

* ensuring agency policy is carried out
* establishing accountability for the work done
* setting priorities and managing workloads
* developing staff knowledge and skills.

Bamford (1982) also saw supervision as a means of ensuring accountability:

> The process of supervision serves ... to reinforce the worker's organisational accountability as well as to facilitate individual development. (p.50)

In social work, supervision can function as a mechanism of accountability and of staff support. Indeed some social workers argue that supervision is more about staff support than about organisational accountability. For example, in their study of area teams, Parsloe and Hill commented on the distinctive social work interpretation of supervision:

> In everyday usage, the word implies a relationship between people in which one has the authority and the responsibility to oversee the work of one or more subordinates... When social workers use the term supervision, they are referring to a process of consultation about cases and methods of work. (1978, paras 8.1 and 8.2)

Williamson (1978) in his study of the probation service found similar views. However, Parsloe and Hill were unequivocal in their rebuttal of this view of supervision:

> Supervision must have two main purposes; to establish the

> accountability of the worker to the organisation and to
> promote the worker's development as a professional person.
> (1978, para. 8.5)

Generally there is agreement in social work that supervision is part of good practice and "the availability of professional supervision is a basic assumption in social work" (Payne, 1977). However, there are important differences between field and residential social work. Field social workers generally receive and are highly satisfied with supervision (Pritchard, 1983). In residential social work, there is no established tradition of supervision and there is agreement that this is detrimental to staff morale and the quality of work (Ward, 1984b, Davies, 1982, Payne, 1977 and Righton, 1985).

Researchers have identified the need for support in residential care. Miller and his colleagues at the Tavistock Institute undertook a series of studies of residential care of people with a disability (Miller and Gwynne, 1971 and Dartington, Miller and Gwynne, 1981). They identified the need for mechanisms of staff support that ensured caring was effectively carried out but did not deny the feelings which it created. As the Wagner Committee has pointed out, caring can be highly demanding, as

> most caring experiences are reciprocal, embodying close
> personal relationships which are frequently bound up with
> powerful and ambivalent feelings of commitment, warmth,
> love, guilt, anxiety, frustration, anger and sometimes
> sexuality. (Wagner Committee, 1988, p.61)

The emotional content of residential care is generated not only by the contact of staff with dependent residents, but also by the daily interaction of staff (see, for example, Dunham, 1978). Douglas and Payne, in an article alleging chronic stress and low morale among many residential staff, quoted a residential social worker's experience of the way in which her work was undermined by lack of continuity, consistency, or even basic co-operation from colleagues:

> It's just a case of whoever is on duty does their own thing,
> and no one agrees with what anyone else is doing. (Douglas
> and Payne, 1985)

Although there is agreement that staff need management

support and that supervision has a crucial role to play in providing this support, there is also the agreement that the field work model of supervision needs to be both modified and supplemented in a residential setting. In a field work setting individual social workers undertake casework with individual clients and supervision can take the form of a face-to-face meeting between the social worker and his or her senior that focuses on the social worker's management of individual cases. Residential social work tends to be more complex. It is a team activity. Groups of staff have to work together to provide care for a group of residents. In this context it is not clear that the prevailing one-to-one model of supervision is adequate.

Payne and Scott (1982) have argued that the one-to-one supervisory relationship is limited not only in the residential setting but also in field work. They argued that decentralisation of field work and the development of community social work have reduced the dependence of field workers on casework models of intervention. Like residential social workers, field workers have become increasingly interdependent and team work is important. They suggested that individual supervision in both field work and residential care needs to be supplemented by team work which focuses on such issues as the allocation of work, the management of resources and the development of staff skills.

Wright (1978), in his discussion of supervision in residential work, also accepted the importance of the team. If supervisors are to provide a role model, then this modelling relationship has to be established within the wider caring group and cannot be confined to a one-to-one encounter. Staff, like residents, need to work out their problems of relating to the group. Wright argued that group work should supplement individual supervision. Individual supervision can provide care staff with personalised support and "time out" from group pressures. Group work can provide staff with the necessary skills to work together creatively and use the caring environment positively.

Just as there is general agreement that individual supervision needs to be linked to group and team dynamics within residential settings, so there is also agreement that the head of a residential unit has a crucial role to play in motivating and supporting staff. According to Miller and Rice (1967) the task of the leader is to maintain staff's commitment to "intrinsically unpleasant, disturbing, or unrewarding activity". The leader must establish credibility in being able to handle the demands placed on staff.

The unit head who remains in the office with the paperwork cannot give this leadership, however regular the supervision sessions he or she offers the staff.

Comment

If small residential units in the community are to create client-centred care, then the role of front-line staff is vital. They provide the bulk of the care and are expected to develop an intensive caring role, often with residents who can provide only limited feedback. The success of these new units depends, to a great extent, on the successful management and support of the front-line care staff.

Within social work, supervision is a major form of staff management and support. Supervision is best developed within field social work, where it fits in well with the dominant form of service provision, individualised case-work. Supervision does exist in residential work, but given the differences in the settings, it needs to be supplemented. The supervisory process needs to be clearly linked to group dynamics through mechanisms such as team meetings. The unit leader will play a crucial model in providing a model for other staff and facilitating positive group relations.

7.2 MECHANISM OF STAFF SUPPORT AND MANAGEMENT

Within Barnardo's all projects, residential and field work, had similar management structures. Each Project had a Project leader who was responsible to an assistant divisional director for the standard of service provided by the Project and for its management. The Project leader was expected to organise a system of meetings so that staff members could discuss the running of the Project and be involved in making decisions. The Project leader was expected to ensure that members of staff received individual support through regular supervision sessions with their line managers.

The divisional managers recognised that the Project leader was central to the success of this Project. He was to play a pivotal role, providing a link between the Project staff and the rest of the Division and between the Project and its environment. He would also ensure that care staff had the resources with which to meet the challenge of caring for the children. In the application to the D.H.S.S. for funds the role and characteristics of the Project leader were described in the following way:

> It is crucial that the occupant of the post of Project Leader possesses the necessary flair, imagination and management ability to ensure the smooth running of the project... The Project Leader will have overall responsibility for the management of the ISU and the staff will be organised in two working groups, one headed by the Deputy, the other by the Third Senior. Each working group will be responsible for the care of one of the sub-groups of four children.

The two working groups model became part of the organisational structure of the Project. Indeed it was reinforced by the physical separation of the two pairs of bungalows. The leader of each working group was given the same status and title of assistant Project leader (A.P.L.). This reinforced the co-ordinating role of Project leader. A deputy could carry out some of the Project leader's functions in his absence, an A.P.L. was more of a Group leader.

The divisional managers recognised that caring for children with a profound mental handicap was demanding. They also accepted that the link worker model required high commitment from care staff. In return divisional managers offered staff involvement in decision-making. This involvement was part of all Barnardo's projects. In the Croxteth Park Project the Project leader wanted staff to feel that through this participation they had an investment in, even an "ownership" of the Project. The Project leader had a key role to play in advising and guiding the staff group but he did not want to impose decisions. For the Project leader staff meetings were more than just a way of transferring information or even of sounding out the opinion of his care staff. They were a form of staff participation. The Project leader described his management style in the following way:

> It's clearly a participative model. Obviously the whole management style of the Project has to take account of the link worker component. The management style recognised the abilities of individuals, no matter what their status, to be part of the creation of internal policies and way of working. That is as long as they had an adequate insight into normalisation... I strove all the way through to get things to come up from the grass roots... It was about giving people an

Staff Management and Support

> ownership, a pride in the thing, a sense of having their ideas and thoughts valued. That doesn't mean you have to accept everything that's thrown up from the grass roots, some things are unworkable. But it does mean that you encourage that creative process, the thoughts and the ideas. You make people feel that they are really involved, not just there to do the "topping and tailing".

Divisional managers recognised that care staff needed support as well as involvement. They felt that each member of care staff should have regular supervision and appraisal. They saw supervision as a regular meeting between Project workers and their immediate line managers to talk in a planned way about work. Staff appraisal was an annual meeting with the line manager to discuss the member of staff's performance and to agree plans for future work. Within the Division, managers preferred to appoint people with a Certification of Qualification in Social Work (C.Q.S.W.) as Project leaders of residential units as they would have experience of supervision and would know how to provide supervision.

Comment

Divisional managers recognised that the Croxteth Park Project was going to be both innovatory and challenging. They were asking care staff to work at the limits of current knowledge and experience and to work in a particular style that would be emotionally demanding and stressful. For the Project to be successful it was vital that staff received adequate support. The Project leader had a central role to play in providing this support. He was the main link between the Project and its environment and he was responsible for ensuring that individuals participated in decision making and received individual supervision.

7.3 SUPPORTING AND MANAGING STAFF

In this section we shall examine the role of the Project leader and his assistants, the Project meetings and supervision in the management and support of the Project staff.

The Role of the Project Leader and his Assistants

The Project leader was primarily a manager. However the Project leader did not define himself as a traditional manager, who concentrated on controlling and directing the activities through a rigid hierarchical system. He saw himself as an enabler, i.e. a person who could create the right conditions for staff and children to interact in a positive and creative way. This particular definition of management affected both his style and particular activities. He emphasised the importance of face-to-face relationships. He wanted to communicate directly with his staff and be involved with them:

> You can sit in an office and send memos. It's one way of ensuring that the job gets done but it's a distant way of operating... It may achieve the task but I have a great anxiety about its effect on morale. People need motivating. It can be a hard, grafting job. It's pretty isolated and lonely if you're grafting away with a couple of kids at 10 o'clock at night. You get a memo... then you go "Oh my God, what do they expect of me". There is a place for the written word but it should really be a confirmation of what has been said.

The emphasis on face-to-face contact permeated the way in which the Project leader operated:

> A lot of my work involves face-to-face contact. Let's talk about the quality of care. That doesn't mean I'm involved in hands-on care but it does involve me in management by walking about... It would involve talking to the children, having coffee and talking to the staff. Just observing general standards, the way the children are dressed, how staff interact, being seen to be part of the thing, sharing news, not being seen as a distant figure, picking up feelings and stress.

The emphasis on staff support also influenced the type of activities the Project leader undertook. He did not see himself as part of a hierarchy. Rather he saw himself as a negotiator or arbitrator who represented both management and the care staff and tried to create mutual understanding.

As the Croxteth Park Project was an experimental Project based on relatively short-term funding, the staff in the Project were conscious that their work was scrutinized and evaluated. Thus an essential part of the Project leader's supportive activity was to manage the relationship between the Project and its wider environment. This involved such activities as dealing with D.H.S.S. inspections and researchers' visits and managing the flow of visitors. Dealing with visitors was especially problematic. On the one hand, divisional managers wanted to make information about the Project available to managers and carers in other agencies and on the other they did not want the children and the staff to be subject to a constant flow of visitors. The Project leader played a crucial role in this area. He limited the number of visitors to the Project and provided alternative sources of information.

To examine the Project leader's role, we asked him to complete a diary of his activities over a period of three weeks during November 1985. We have divided the Project leader's activities into four broad categories, administration, e.g. dealing with correspondence, preparing budgets; managing and supporting staff, e.g. staff supervision; managing relations with the agency, e.g. meeting with the assistant divisional director; and relating to the wider environment, e.g. meeting D.H.S.S. inspectors. The Project leader had a very busy work schedule. Excluding travelling the Project leader worked nearly 40 hours per week. The Project leader's priorities clearly influenced his allocation of time. He spent most time managing and supervising his staff (over 48 hours, 40% total time). Indeed, staff supervision was the single most time-consuming activity (34 hr. 30 min. or nearly 30% of total time). The second most important activity in terms of time allocation was relating to other managers in the agency (35 hr. 30 min. or 30% of total time). The third most important was managing relations with the environment (18 hr. 30 min. or just over 15% of total time). The Project leader allocated the smallest amount of his time to traditional administrative activities (16 hr 55 min or 14% of total time).

The Project leader took overall managerial responsibility for the Project and acted as the main link with the agency and the environment. He was supported in this work by two assistant Project leaders. The A.P.L.s in particular helped with the internal management of the Project. They dealt with many of the day-to-day administrative activities. Each A.P.L. provided leadership for one staff group. As first line managers they were on the management/care interface and they had an administrative and caring role.

In practice the A.P.L.s found it difficult to reconcile the caring

Staff Management and Support

and administrative functions. In Phase One, the staff experimented with different staff rotas. In one rota, the administrative and caring time of the A.P.L. were separated. In the other, they were not and the A.P.L. had to make decisions on allocation of time on a day-to-day basis. In Phase Two, the staff developed a six-week rota in which the A.P.L. worked with each of the R.S.W.s for a period. Whatever pattern of working was adopted, there was considerable pressure on the A.P.L. to be involved in child care. As a result all the A.P.L.s tended to work extra hours to complete their administrative activities.

Group Processes

An important part of the internal management of the Project were the various meetings held in the Project. We shall concentrate on the two main types of meetings, staff meetings and group meetings.

Staff Meetings formed the main link between the staff in the Project and the rest of the Division. They were held once a month and chaired by the Project leader. They were formal meetings for which written agendas were circulated beforehand and written minutes circulated afterwards. The staff agreed to have separate staff meetings for each phase because of the problems of staff availability.

The Project leader set the agendas and chaired the meetings, which lasted about an hour and a half. The Project leader used the meeting to report back on the various committees which he had attended and to keep Project staff informed of the changes in agency policy. For example, at a joint staff meeting of both phases of the Project held in July 1984, 22 items were discussed. All of them were introduced by the Project leader. This particular meeting was atypical. At most meetings staff raised issues for discussion, e.g. specific children or care issues. For example, in a meeting held in Phase One in May 1984, the Project leader reported back on a discussion that was held at the divisional manager's meeting on male staff caring for female children. The Project staff used this opportunity to raise the issue of Margaret the oldest girl in the Project who was reaching puberty. This sort of discussion was fairly exceptional in staff meetings and when specific issues were raised, the Project leader tended to refer them to the group meetings.

Like most residential workers, Project staff did not appear to like staff meetings very much. They felt that these meetings tended to be a monologue given by the Project leader and that issues that interested and concerned them were not really discussed. The Project leader was aware of these problems and tried to increase the participation of staff in these meetings. For example, he invited staff to submit items for the agenda but generally they did not. Like many carers, the staff were immersed in the practicalities of caring and found it difficult to see an overall context for their personalised caring work.

Group Meetings Each phase held a weekly group meeting of about an hour chaired by the A.P.L. These were less formal than the staff meetings which dealt with the operation of each phase and team relationships. There were fixed subjects for discussion, e.g. the children and goal planning, and additional topics were agreed at the start of each meeting. The Project leader generally did not attend these meetings. He read the minutes.

The main focus of the group meetings was the practical organisation of the day-to-day care. Issues such as rotas, division of tasks were regularly discussed. Another important function of the group meetings was to complement supervision and discuss team functioning. The Project leader wanted staff to discuss team dynamics and the normalisation philosophy, but staff in both phases found this sort of generalised discussion very difficult. Discussions of group dynamics tended to occur in supervision.

Team relations were sometimes discussed in terms of Phase One versus Phase Two. Senior management had hoped at the inception of the Project that dividing the Project into two phases would not create competition between the two phases. However, once the Project was under way everyone accepted that this was inevitable. Certainly up to the beginning of 1985 staff in Phase Two felt that there was an unequal relationship between the two phases. The secretary and the project office were housed in Phase One and the Project leader operated in Phase One as an A.P.L. for a time. At a Phase Two group meeting in October 1985, some frustrations were voiced about their perception of receiving less information and support from the Project leader, and staff said that they felt like the "poorer relations".

Staff did raise some policy issues at group meetings. For example, in Phase One, there was a series of group meetings that raised, in the autumn of 1984, issues about the general management and operation of the Project. In the meeting of 3rd September 1984 there was a discussion of professional input and use of resources. This discussion raised several general issues about the operation of the Project. For example:

> * A general point was made about the autonomy of R.S.W.s to take the initiative and make decisions about the children's development without receiving criticism from management after the decision had been made ...
> * There was general agreement within the group of the need to listen to what the Project leader said "on the side" on normalisation and the need to discuss it in the light of what professionals had to offer in the development of each child, (e.g. whether a 12 year old should be fed with a plastic baby spoon).

These issues then formed the basis for subsequent discussions with the Project leader.

The role of the A.P.L.s was central to the group meetings. Each A.P.L. defined the role differently. In 1985 the A.P.L. in Phase One was particularly concerned about the care tasks and standards of care. This sometimes placed her in an explicit inspectorial role and set her apart from the group. The A.P.L. in Phase Two brought these issues up within a wider discussion of the children, communication or practical arrangements between staff. It seemed that this method was more effective. The difference in style had been noted by the Project leader and he initiated discussions with the A.P.L. from Phase One about her management style. This A.P.L. left the Project in December 1985 and many of the issues remained unresolved. The lessons learned, however, were valuable for the next appointment of an A.P.L. as it had become increasingly clear that the A.P.L.s played a pivotal role in the daily operation of the Project.

Supervision

There was a range of one-to-one meetings in the Project. They varied in formality and frequency from the annual appraisal meeting in which members of staff met with their line managers to discuss their job performance, through formal supervision meetings that took place at least once a month, through to informal supervision that sometimes took place daily. In this section we shall concentrate on the formal supervision sessions as these were a distinctive feature of the Project.

Within the Project, the Project leader introduced a fieldwork model of supervision. He supervised the two A.P.L.s, who in turn each supervised five R.S.W.s. The formal supervisions were private meetings. The participants made appointments to meet at regular intervals. At the start of the meeting they agreed an agenda for discussion and at the end they prepared a record of the meeting. The records of the meetings were kept in a separate file to which the participants had access.

Project Leader/A.P.L. The Project leader provided his A.P.L.s with regular formal supervision sessions. He provided a formal session of at least one hour at least once a fortnight. He supplemented this with shorter informal sessions when there were matters requiring immediate attention. In one three-week period we sampled the Project leader provided his A.P.L.s with four formal supervision sessions, each took approximately two hours, and six informal sessions. These informal sessions tended to last 45 minutes, though one session lasted four hours.

We analysed the topics covered in a sample of 17 formal supervision sessions. It was possible to classify the topics covered in the same broad categories we used to analyse the activities of the Project leader. The balance of the issues was different. Whereas the Project leader spent over 45% of his time managing relations between the Project and its environment, only 14% of the topics covered in supervision involved these issues. As might be expected the overwhelming majority of topics covered in supervision dealt with the administration and management of the Project and in particular staff relations. Over 40% of the topics covered in supervision concerned relations between staff and staffing issues.

Generally the supervision sessions focused on the needs of the A.P.L.s. The A.P.L.s prepared for the supervision session by listing the topics they wanted to discuss. The Project leader defined his role as providing guidance and support. He usually responded to the issues raised by the A.P.L.s. As the only member of staff with a C.Q.S.W. qualification and with previous experience of supervision, the Project leader saw himself as providing a model which the A.P.L. could then use as the basis of their role as supervisors.

A.P.L./R.S.W. There are variations in the ways in which different A.P.L.s interpreted their role as supervisors. At the time we were conducting our research rather different patterns had developed in the two Phases. This was partly related to the different histories of the two Phases. In Phase One there were relatively long periods during which the A.P.L. post was vacant, e.g. November 1984 until April 1985. R.S.W.s in Phase One tended to have periods during which they received fortnightly formal supervision from an A.P.L. alternating with periods during which they received supervision every four or five weeks from the Project leader. In Phase Two, R.S.W.s tended to receive regular monthly supervision from their A.P.L.

The focus of the supervision sessions in both phases was on child care and the caring process. In neither phase were any wider issues such as relations with the agency or relations with the wider environment discussed. There was some discussion of general administration but compared to the discussion in the P.L./A.P.L. supervision this was only a minor topic. Only three of the 10 R.S.W.s said they frequently discussed general administrative issues. The supervision in Phase One was more task centred and the A.P.L. tended to initiate discussion about team dynamics. In Phase Two there was more emphasis on staff support with the A.P.L. raising issues related to the caring process such as R.S.W.s' feelings or subjective response to care and the nature of the skills required to provide care.

Comment

The divisional managers developed a comprehensive and formal system for managing and supporting staff in the Project. This system involved clearly defined management structures and relationships, a clearly defined process of decision-making involving staff participation and a system of staff supervision.

In terms of management structures, the Project leader had clear management responsibility for the Project. He was a full-time manager who was accountable to an assistant divisional director for the overall performance of the Project. Although the Project leader devoted the majority of his time to "managing" the Project, he did not see himself as a traditional manager. He minimised the amount of traditional office-based administration and concentrated on supporting his staff through personal contact. A major part of his role was linking and managing the relations between the Project and its environment.

The Project leader wanted to encourage staff involvement. He did this in two ways by delegating the day-to-day running of the Project to his assistants and by involving the staff in decision-making. The care staff were expected to take part not only in decisions that affected the Project but also to contribute to debates that affected the agency's national policy. They did this through the medium of staff and group meetings.

To help staff cope with the demands of caring, the Project had a system of regular supervision. Members of staff had the right to receive regular and confidential supervision from their line managers. Each member of staff had the right to raise any issue related to the operation of the Project and the provision of care.

7.4 ASSESSING STAFF MANAGEMENT AND SUPPORT

In this section we shall examine the effectiveness of the various mechanisms adopted by the Project to manage and support staff. We shall discuss each mechanism in turn.

Management Roles and Relations

The Project leader had a key role to play in the management of the Project. The Division was fortunate to be able to appoint an experienced, professionally qualified and highly committed person as Project leader. He was able to provide professional and managerial leadership and to act as a role model for the carers in the Project. His style of leadership was clearly imprinted on the Project. The Project leader had the confidence and the support of divisional managers.

The Project leader's role was highly demanding and stressful. As a middle manager, he was in many senses a "piggy in the middle". When the care staff felt under stress then their anxieties tended to focus on the Project leader. He could at times come to represent an unfriendly, even hostile environment, e.g. the Division which "refused" to provide care staff with the extra resources they required. Thus when the Project was under stress, and this was particularly the case during the first winter, the Project leader was subjected to criticism, particularly by the care staff. However, when the Project was running smoothly, the Project leader did not necessarily get the credit. For example, the successful implementation of a goal plan tended to be credited to the link worker.

The middle management role of the Project leader was reflected in the type of job satisfaction he received. It was satisfaction derived from establishing the right conditions for

Staff Management and Support

other people to deliver care:

> My satisfaction comes from seeing children develop and enjoying life, hearing David singing when he wakes up in the morning... It's probably greater satisfaction for link workers but it gives me a kick... It gives me satisfaction to see staff develop, whether this is because they have moved on to some kind of training or they have developed in the Project and have something to offer. I get satisfaction from a sense of personal investment in the kids and staff, about the kind of ethos that exists in the Project. You are trying to prove something, trying to develop an openness and a welcoming atmosphere, where parents feel comfortable and secure.

Senior divisional managers were successful in appointing an experienced social worker as Project leader who had developed a positive style of management. They were less successful with the A.P.L. posts. Problems in attracting suitable people for this post emerged at the very start of the Project. The divisional managers appointed a well-qualified person to be A.P.L. in Phase One but she withdrew at a late stage so that the staff group in the first phase did not have an A.P.L. during their training and preparation period. Generally divisional managers dealt with the A.P.L. problem by either considering applicants who had applied for R.S.W. posts or by internal promotions of R.S.W.s who seemed to have management skills. They had successes and also some clear failures.

A.P.L.s had to provide leadership to their staff group by example, i.e. they were involved in child care, but they also had to provide clear management guidance through group meetings and staff supervision. The A.P.L.s generally found it difficult to balance these two activities and tended to emphasise the child care aspects. For example, it was the A.P.L.s' role to encourage and to acknowledge the individual efforts of staff but they had on occasion neglected to do this, especially in the early stages of the Project. Similarly it was the A.P.L.s' responsibility to function as a link between their staff group and the whole Project. As the A.P.L.s had tended not to do this a degree of tension and competition had developed between the two staff groups. One consequence of the shortcomings of the A.P.L.s was that it increased the pressure on the Project leader. At one stage this was formalised when the Project leader temporarily took on the role of A.P.L. in Phase One. The failure of the A.P.L.s in the early stage to develop a managerial role meant there was a tendency for a polarisation to develop between "carers" and "managers".

Divisional managers accepted that the A.P.L. role was vital for the operation of the Project and that it had not been developed successfully in the early stages of the Project. They felt that much of the responsibility lay with national policies. As the Wagner Committee (1988) has pointed out, there is "no overall body which is charged with workforce planning" (p.71) in residential care. Therefore there is no national programme of staff development and training for this type of post. Furthermore, in social work terms, the A.P.L. post is seen as having relatively low status and does not fit into a well-developed career structure. In view of national problems, the Division decided to develop its own programme in basic managerial skills for group leaders. The first course was held in 1986.

Group Processes

The Project leader acknowledged that it had taken time to develop a culture of participation:

> The process of decision-making worked pretty well... It was not perfect initially, it took a bit of time to develop... People didn't really expect it, they weren't accustomed to it... Initially they were unsure and suspicious, they were not sure what they had to offer. They were overwhelmed by the anxiety of having responsibility for the care of the kids, initially they were overwhelmed. They were suspicious of tokenism... People gradually overcame their suspicions when it was demonstrated that they did have a say; they were allowed to plan their own rotas as long as management was sure that the rota provided satisfactory cover; they could create a system they felt comfortable with.

The Project staff did not have such positive attitudes. They accepted participation that resulted in quick decisions and visible results. For example, the care staff all had positive attitudes towards group meetings. They felt they could discuss issues at these meetings that related to their immediate concerns and they could, through these discussions, make decisions. However care staff were less positive about contributing to general policy and to staff meetings. When we first talked to care staff about staff meetings in 1984, they clearly did not like these meetings. They felt that these meetings concentrated on matters such as Divisional Managers' meetings which did not interest them. In 1985 the Project leader undertook a major review of staff meetings. He accepted the importance of communicating agency policy to care staff but decided to collate some of the material in written form. The Project leader decided to focus on specific issues that were of importance to the Project at each meeting. At the November meeting he focused on the "life long care" issue. As this was a major concern to Project staff, they did contribute to the discussion, and the Project leader was able to identify issues to bring to the attention of the Barnardo's working party discussing the issue.

The care staff were, at times, unclear about the limits of their participation in decision-making. These problems can be clearly seen in discussions on child selection. In October 1984 there was a lengthy discussion at a Phase One group meeting about the selection of a child. The staff felt that they had not been sufficiently involved in the decision-making process. They felt that they were expected to care for a child who had been selected by managers. As "hands-on" carers they felt they should have been consulted as a group. The Project leader was clear that the final responsibility for the decision lay with the managers as they had to reconcile divergent and at times conflicting interests. However he did acknowledge the importance of consulting care staff and initiated special group meetings to discuss the selection of children. Two such meetings took place in November and December 1985 and they clearly gave staff a sense of shared responsibility and involvement in decision-making.

Supervision

In view of the patchy provision of supervision in residential settings, a major success of the Project, was that each member of staff received regular formal supervision. Each member of staff had the opportunity to discuss their work and to identify any areas in which they wanted advice and support.

Generally the staff in the Project found supervision helpful. We interviewed the two A.P.L.s in 1985 and they both found supervision an invaluable support for their activities as managers. They used supervision as a major means of communication and of assessing their performance. The two A.P.L.s used supervision in

Staff Management and Support

different ways. The A.P.L. in Phase One was, at the time of the interview, relatively new to the job and she used supervision as a way of gaining advice and guidance about the management of her group. She saw it as a mechanism of personal support and development. The A.P.L. in Phase Two was established in her post. She recognised that the Project leader was willing, even keen, to offer personal support but did not feel she needed such support. She used supervision as a way of discussing specific tasks and decisions. Although both A.P.L.s used supervision in different ways both said they felt comfortable in supervision and both felt they could express their views, even when they disagreed with their supervisor.

However there were costs. The Project leader and the A.P.L.s commented that it took time to build up a relationship of confidence and trust and they were short of time. This was a particular problem for the A.P.L.s who had a caring role and a number of R.S.W.s to supervise. In Phase Two, the staff adopted a rota which "protected" some of the A.P.L.s' time for activities such as supervision. In Phase One the rotas did not specifically "protect" time. As the A.P.L. gave priority to care, she tended to provide supervision outside her normal duty time.

The R.S.W.s generally found supervision useful. Eight of the 10 R.S.W.s we interviewed said they found supervision a useful way of communicating and in particular they used it to check on their progress, to gain advice and guidance and to discuss specific issues that were causing them problems. One R.S.W. commented that he found supervision a better medium than group meetings for solving problems. Only two R.S.W.s did not find supervision helpful. Both said they found it too slow to solve problems. They said they tended to solve problems informally and then use the supervision session to get formal approval.

There were some differences between R.S.W.s' experience of supervision. R.S.W.s in Phase One saw supervision as important but they tended to emphasise a task-oriented form of supervision. Thus Phase One R.S.W.s tended to see supervision as important because "it keeps you on your toes" and "management knows your progress". In Phase Two the R.S.W.s had the opportunity to build up a supportive relationship with their A.P.L. and in their interviews tended to discuss supervision in terms such as "trust, confidence, respect, guidance and support". They tended to see supervision as important because "you have time alone", "you can organise your thoughts" and "it's important for communication".

Comment

Senior divisional managers had developed a sophisticated system of staff support and management. This system functioned well. However there were problems and costs. The roles of both the Project leader and the A.P.L.s were difficult and stressful. The agency was fortunate in being able to recruit a high-calibre Project leader but his job was made more stressful by inadequate support from A.P.L.s. There was no ready-made pool of first-line managers which the division could draw on. The division had to train its own. In the short term this created problems.

Participatory decision-making was time consuming for both managers and care staff. Managers had to spend time listening to staff while care staff had to take the trouble to consider the issues. Care staff were more willing to make the necessary investment when they felt that the issues involved their immediate work environment. They found it more difficult to be involved in more general long-term policy discussions. It was to the credit of the Project leader that he persisted in raising such issues.

Supervision was an important mechanism of staff support. Although supervisors could not "solve" all their supervisees' problems, supervision offered carers an opportunity to articulate their problems and needs and a way of drawing on the advice and experience of their line managers.

7.5 SUMMARY AND COMMENT

Staff are the major and key resource of any residential project. Managers need to manage and support care staff to ensure that the residents receive a satisfactory quality of care and to see that the staff are not exhausted or damaged in the process.

Within social work, supervision forms a major mechanism of staff management and support. Supervision has tended to develop within a field-work setting where the one-to-one relationship between a field social worker and his or her supervisor mirrors and fits in well with the dominant case work model of field work. However this model of supervision does not fit as well to other models of field work, e.g. community work, nor does it fit as well with other settings such as residential social work. In these instances supervision needs to be supplemented by other forms of management and support.

Staff Management and Support

In the Croxteth Park Project, the divisional managers accepted the central role of the care staff in achieving the objectives of the Project. They acknowledged that they were making high demands of their staff and in exchange they expected to provide staff with good quality managerial support. As part of a social work agency, the Division drew on social work practice, in particular they accepted that the Project leader and his assistants had a key role to play in managing the internal relations of the Project and linking the Project to its environment. They expected the Project leader and his assistants to provide leadership through collective mechanisms, such as staff meetings, and individual mechanisms, such as supervision.

The divisional managers were fortunate to be able to appoint a professionally qualified social worker as Project leader. The Project leader was committed both to the principles of normalisation and to participatory styles of management. The Project leader provided a strong model for his assistants and for the R.S.W.s. He sought to give staff an involvement and ownership in the Project and the children.

There can be no doubt that the Project leader was extremely successful in generating commitment to the children. However there were costs and limitations. The Project leader's own role was highly stressful and, because of the underdevelopment of the A.P.L. role, he received relatively little support. The participatory style of leadership was time consuming, both for the Project leader and for the care staff. Both managers and care staff had to be willing to invest time in building relations and participating in decisions. When care staff could see the immediate benefits they were willing to do so, but when the benefits were not so obvious they were not.

8 RELATIVES, NEIGHBOURS AND VOLUNTEERS: MOBILISING THE INFORMAL SECTOR OF CARE

ANNE CHAPPELL AND ANDY ALASZEWSKI

The informal sector has always played a major part in providing care and support for dependent people. The development of care in the community policies has highlighted the role of this sector. Care in institutions is provided by staff. The physical isolation of most institutions means that they can only make limited use of the informal sector. Care based in the community has greater potential for developing this wider range of support. In this chapter we discuss the nature of the informal sector and the ways in which Barnardo's mobilised this wider support.

8.1 DEFINING AND USING THE INFORMAL SECTOR

The government accepts that informal care is an essential part of community care and has advised welfare agencies that they should support, mobilise and supplement informal care:

> the informal sector is vital to community based care and needs to be sustained and strengthened...it is important not to assume that the amount of informal care can be limitlessly increased. The organised voluntary sector and statutory agencies must aim to supplement natural networks where these are deficient. (D.H.S.S., 1981e, p.48)

However, there are many difficulties when formal agencies attempt to incorporate the informal sector into their care provision. One difficulty is trying to define the precise nature of the informal sector. It is hard to provide exact definitions because informal care is characterised by its variability and the way in which its patterns of provision merge into each other.

There are no clear boundaries between one form of informal care and another. The D.H.S.S. has argued

> it is important to distinguish between the different components of the voluntary sector. A broad classification runs from informal carers (family, friends and neighbours) through mutual aid groups, neighbourhood care groups and volunteers to formally constituted voluntary organisations. (D.H.S.S., 1981e, p.48)

Informal care is unpredictable; what one neighbour may see as helpfulness another may see as intrusion. It is sporadic; care may be offered regularly, occasionally or never. It is frequently mobilised in times of crises, for example, after the death of a family member.

There is evidence that the structure of the informal sector is undergoing significant change. Friendship is a new source of informal support for many people. Abrams has argued there are now two informal care systems. There is a traditional form based on

> a densely woven world of kin, neighbours, friends and co-workers, highly localized and strongly caring within the confines of quite tightly defined relationships, above all the relationships of kinship. (Abrams, 1984, p.414)

This is the informal system identified by Young and Willmott (1957) in their study of Bethnal Green, East London. The second system identified by Abrams is characterised by friendship, i.e. relations built on choice rather than constraint.

There is general agreement that informal networks are beneficial to the well-being of society. They indicate that people care about and for each other. However there are some drawbacks. Abrams (1977) has pointed out that communities with an extensive development of traditional forms of informal support are almost always communities which suffer from industrial decline and deprivation. Moreover, communities with large immigrant populations may have well-developed patterns of mutual support (Abrams, 1977), but this may mean that the community members see each other as the only sources of support and welfare. They may view the statutory agencies as hostile or disinterested and, therefore their informal networks maybe a sign of isolation from the rest of society.

Most mentally handicapped people live with their families (D.H.S.S., 1980). Family care may include support from other sources, such as the extended family, neighbours, friends or the statutory authorities. At different times there may be different combinations of carers, although the overwhelming burden of care remains with women in the family. It is not the community that cares for vulnerable or dependent people but their close female relatives (see, for example, Ayer and Alaszewski, 1986). However to continue to expect women to be willing or able to provide the core of informal care is "a very shaky basis on which to plan the expansion of community care" (Finch and Groves, 1980, p.506). Social changes are reducing the availability of women. For example, families have fewer children so the chance of finding an adult child to care for an aged parent has been reduced; families do not always live near their kin; women are increasingly economically active and traditional caring obligations are becoming blurred by increasing cohabitation, divorce and remarriage (Finch and Groves, 1980).

The word "community" implies warmth and a caring relationship. Yet it may be neither of these things if the community is non-existent except in a literal, physical sense. If the community does not wish to care for its members then people discharged from hospital may be placed in other institutions such as nursing homes, residential homes or prisons. The Social Services Committee described the "dumping" of mentally ill or mentally handicapped people in prisons as "a mockery of community care" (Social Services Committee, 1985).

If community-based units are to be different from hospitals then they must find effective ways of mobilising informal care. Surprisingly, there are few studies of the ways in which the informal sector can be mobilised so that it participates in the care provision for people in the community with handicaps and disabilities. Shearer, in a review of innovatory services stressed that these services were all

> committed to enabling people with mental handicaps and their families to share in the ordinary life of their communities. (Shearer, 1986, p.12)

However she drew attention to the findings of a survey of 35 people with a mental handicap living independently in Avon which "found that isolation and loneliness remain a major problem" (p.128). She argued that "to live in the community is not automatically to be part of it" (p.129).

Atkinson and Ward (1987) have undertaken one of the few studies which examines the relations established by people discharged from hospital. They interviewed 50 people who had left hospital to live in different parts of Somerset. Atkinson and Ward argued:

> the quality of their lives was, to a great extent, determined by the range and type of their social relationships. They described their lives and lifestyles in terms of the people they knew - the people they shared house with, members of their family, their friends and workmates, and people in their neighbourhood. (p.232)

Several people experienced social isolation but the majority had well-established and fruitful relationships. They had achieved community acceptance and five had even developed community participation (p. 241). Atkinson and Ward argued that

> we have been slow to realise that helping people settle into ordinary houses in ordinary streets does not of itself bring integration into the "community" or a high quality of life. For that, we have to look beyond bricks and mortar, to ways of encouraging the development of social relationships in community settings. (p. 242)

8.2 USING THE INFORMAL SECTOR OF CARE

The senior divisional managers saw the Project as a way of providing institutionalised children with experiences of normal life rather than a social experiment in which the children were integrated into the "community". For example, divisional managers described the role of volunteers in the initial application to the D.H.S.S. in the following way:

> The volunteers should make a unique contribution to the work of the ISU by broadening the range of experiences to which the children are exposed, and in building links between the unit and the local community. (Barnardo's, 1981c, p.10)

Relatives, Neighbours and Volunteers

To provide children with normal social relations and experiences, the Division wanted to develop a network of social support for the children and the Project. The link workers were to act as surrogate parents for the children and, if the bonding worked, this relationship would provide each child with a significant relationship with an adult. Barnardo's wanted to provide each child with other relationships that children living in a family might experience, such as with relatives, friends and neighbours.

Initially the working group considered using formal community organisations such as self-help groups and community groups as a way of gaining access to the informal sector. However, as they collected more information about the nature of local groups, their principal interest shifted to developing relationships with individuals:

> We didn't tie into voluntary groups... Not that we didn't want to contribute, we did... My personal view is that they didn't have anything to offer the kids. They might have something to offer in terms of Barnardo's image, giving it a higher profile in the area... There were one or two groups, not many.

The divisional managers felt that they could better develop relationships for the children by enhancing the children's existing links with the relatives of the children, recruiting volunteers and developing positive relations with neighbours.

Families

Barnardo's has clear agency policies for families. When children are in residential care, Barnardo's seeks to involve their parents in the caring process, for example, by encouraging visits. Where possible the residential project should be a reasonable distance from the family home to "facilitate parental visits" (Barnardo's, 1968, p.14).

The divisional managers wanted to encourage the children's families to participate in the Project and develop a close relationship with their child. Parents were seen as key people in the children's lives. The Division wanted the parents, as far as possible, to participate in the decision making and in the day-to-day life of the children.

Neighbours

Barnardo's believe that the children in its care will benefit from care in a community environment. This implies some degree of interaction between projects and the community.

The divisional managers wanted to encourage the involvement of neighbours through a "good neighbour" policy. The care staff would be the first point of contact between the Project and the community. It was vital that the Project was staffed with people who were able to form good relationships with neighbours. These staff needed to avoid antagonising neighbours and to appear friendly. In order to establish friendships with the neighbours, the divisional managers recognised that it was not sufficient for the staff to be merely receptive to their neighbours. They would also have to be willing to go out and establish contact. This would involve helping other people move into their houses, holding house-warming parties and maintaining friendly relations after everyone had settled down in the estate. The Project developed an "open house" policy and tried to make neighbours feel able to drop into the project to look around and have a chat. The Project staff felt that the usual tacit "rules" between neighbours of non-interference and privacy should not be applied strictly. The R.S.W.s had to be active in achieving good relations with the community to overcome people's "fear" of mental handicap and to give the children opportunities to interact with the informal sector. They welcomed any interest from neighbours, as long as it was not damaging or degrading to the children.

Volunteers

Barnardo's attached great importance to the use of volunteers in its projects.

> The Agency also sees itself fulfilling a philanthropic role by recruiting volunteers, because it provides them with an opportunity to express their caring for their fellow man in an emotional and practical way. (Barnardo's, 1981b, para.4.2)

Barnardo's believes that its clients benefit from volunteers:

> we are effectively opening up our doors to the outside and allowing a healthy inter-change between our clients and the

Relatives, Neighbours and Volunteers

community. (Barnardo's, 1981b, para.4.2)

Barnardo's volunteers undergo a selection procedure and enter a contractual agreement with the agency and are, therefore, to some degree accountable. Barnardo's do not see volunteers as an alternative or substitute to be used when a project is short-staffed, but expect volunteers to develop a distinctive role within each project.

In the Croxteth Park Project divisional managers felt that volunteers had an important role to play in complementing the work of staff. They saw volunteers as having a significant role to play in developing relations with children and by cooperating with paid staff in carrying out the children's programmes. Divisional managers wanted to recruit 24 volunteers so that each child could develop relations with 3 volunteers.

Comment

The Project staff accepted that the informal sector has an important role to play in providing the children with the normal experiences of everyday life. The planning group initially considered using formal organisations to develop these relations but decided that it was more fruitful to develop relations with individuals.

8.3 RELATING TO THE INFORMAL SECTOR

Divisional managers stressed the importance of the attitudes of care staff in the establishment and enhancement of the children's relationship with their relatives, neighbours and volunteers. In the staff training programme, managers devoted sessions to building up positive attitudes amongst the care staff so that they valued the contribution of the informal sector.

Parents

The involvement of parents in the Project was a priority and started when the children were first considered for the Project. Field social workers visited the parents of all children considered for the Project to discuss it. The divisional managers wanted parents to have enough information to make a real decision:

> One reason for visiting the parents is to make sure they really agree to the child moving. At no point would that be done without that approval. It is also to give them information, reassure them and allay fears... If the parents said they were not interested that would be their decision.

The divisional managers felt that proper field social work was essential in increasing and maintaining the parents' confidence. Initially they used the hospital social workers but found that the hospital social workers did not provide an adequate service. In particular they tended to avoid sensitive issues and provided a token service once the child had been admitted to the Project:

> We found that things we felt should have been spelt out hadn't been. The hospital social workers hadn't talked through substantial parts of the proposal such as possible foster placements. Some of the issues had been avoided because of high emotional content... We realised that to ensure that it was done properly we would have to do it ourselves. In one of the later cases all the information the parents received was a short letter, very brief. It said something to the effect that "Your child has been selected for this new Barnardo's facility. We are confident that it would be in his best interest to go. Your child will be transferred on such and such a date. If you want to talk about this 'phone me." This was not the way we wanted to work with parents. We stopped the process. We had a planning meeting. We said that at the very least they needed an explanation of what was going on. The Project Leader went to visit the family and worked with them until we got a part-time social worker.

Project staff wanted to make parents feel that they were an important part of the planning process. Parents were consulted on issues concerning their child, for example over matters of medical treatment. They were always invited to the six-monthly reviews and were encouraged to participate in discussion on their child's future but the Project leader recognised that

> Some parents can't cope with the relationship. They have little contact if any. Even in those cases something can develop. Take Stuart's case. Following my initial visit, mum actually started to come, she hadn't had any contact for 7 years. O.K., she only came to review meetings but she was involved in planning his future. That was all she could cope with but at least she had the opportunity.

The role of the link workers was central in developing relations with the family. They took on responsibility for maintaining contact with the family. When the family visited they were usually met by the link worker who tried to make them feel welcome, even if this involved using resources, e.g. for the provision of refreshments. The staff wanted to encourage spontaneity. When one child's extended family came to visit without prior warning, the staff considered it a great compliment that the family should feel sufficiently comfortable in the Project to visit their child when they wanted to. The Project leader described the role of link workers in the following way:

> Everybody's responsible for making the parents feel welcome so that they feel comfortable and can drop in at any time. The link worker will model (sic) by valuing the parents and their contribution to their child's life.

One objective of the Project was to find fostering placements for some of the children. The role of the fostering team was to find suitable foster parents and gradually familiarise the child with his or her new home and foster family. Barnardo's was conscious that its commitment to family life for the children might cause some problems. Some of the natural parents did not realise that fostering was such an important objective in the Project when they agreed to the transfer of their child. The fostering team reassured the parents that fostering would only proceed with their consent and that they could maintain contact with their child after fostering. Some of the children had a close relationship with their natural parents and fostering was not a major objective for these children.

Neighbours

When the Project was in its planning stages, there was some hostility among other residents of the estate. The divisional managers decided not to accept an invitation from the residents' association to discuss the Project as they felt this would give a platform to a hostile minority:

> We had some problems on the estate when people started to find out that we were setting up a Project on Croxteth Park. All sorts of rumours were going round saying Barnardo's were going to place juvenile delinquents on the estate. We

> decided not to formally reply to the tenants' association or any other organisation on the estate as we did not want to make an issue out of it. We wanted to be able to move in like Mrs. Johnson next door. We have a right to buy a house and move in like anybody else.

The Project did make some use of semi-formal organisations to develop relations with the community. For example, the staff of Phase Two became active participants of the local residents' association. They also volunteered to take part in a Neighbourhood Watch Scheme. Burglaries were fairly common on the estate and the Project always had a member of staff awake on duty. Attempts to use semi-formal organisations were not always successful. For example, the staff wanted some of the older children to join local Girl Guide and Boy Scout groups. These applications were turned down at first, but the Project staff persevered.

The children were taken into the neighbourhood as much as possible, involved in everyday pursuits. They were taken shopping and for walks. As far as possible, the R.S.W.s used normal facilities for the children. They travelled in taxis rather than ambulances and went to the hairdressers, rather than having a home visit. The children wore attractive clothes and the R.S.W.s tried to discourage gifts of second-hand clothes or toys from neighbours.

The Project staff were particularly concerned to develop relations with their immediate neighbours. Phase One was one of six pairs of bungalows in a small cul-de-sac on the estate. Barnardo's moved in after the other neighbours. The staff held a house-warming party to establish contact with its neighbours. Project staff tried to help their neighbours. For example, Project staff telephoned the fire brigade when a neighbour's house caught fire and they helped clear out a neighbour's kitchen when it flooded.

Phase Two bungalows were at a T-junction on the main road through the estate. There was always activity outside the Project and many people to talk to. The Project moved in before the other neighbours and so staff were able to offer help to the neighbours when they moved in. The staff also held a house-warming party which gave an opportunity for all the new neighbours to introduce themselves.

Volunteers

The process for selecting and training the first group of volunteers was modelled on the process of selection and training of the staff, especially the R.S.W.s. Indeed, in the application for funds to the D.H.S.S., volunteers were discussed under the heading "Staff Training" and there were explicit parallels between the volunteers and the staff:

> Whilst accepting that staff and volunteers have specific and distinctive training, the Project will identify certain training elements which could be carried out together.

The selection process of the staff and volunteers had the same elements. The Division advertised for volunteers, took up references and interviewed volunteers and gave them a similar, but shorter, training programme. There were also important differences. Divisional managers wanted to recruit more volunteers than staff, and they had less tangible rewards to offer volunteers. They could offer them travelling expenses but the main reward was the intrinsic satisfaction of volunteering. The volunteers operated under the supervision of the staff, especially the R.S.W.s, and their access to the children was controlled by the R.S.W.s. For example, the volunteers did not meet the children during their training period as Project staff felt that the children were not "on show". Instead the volunteers received written descriptions of each child. During the training programme, the trainers established hierarchical relations between the care staff and the volunteers.

The role of the volunteers in the Project was also modelled on that of the staff. Indeed, divisional managers wanted the first group of staff and the first group of volunteers to start work at the same time so that they could learn together and develop complementary roles. One example of this explicit modelling was the development of visiting rotas. The Project staff felt that, like staff, volunteers should attend regularly and therefore in discussions with the volunteers, they arranged a rota of visits. At the beginning of each week a member of staff telephoned all volunteers to confirm their visits.

Comment

The Project aimed to enhance the children's relationships by developing contact with relatives, neighbours and volunteers. The individuals in each of these categories had a different relationship to the Project, so the Project staff adopted a different approach to each group. Parents were given the most support and had the most scope in choosing how to relate to the Project. The Project staff saw their relationship with the children as vitally important to the success of the Project and also recognised the sensitivity of the relationship. The Project staff related to the neighbours through their good neighbour policy. They consciously avoided being a nuisance and also identified ways in which the Project could be a positive asset to the neighbourhood. The Project tended to treat volunteers as complementary to the staff and initially developed a formal process for recruiting, training and defining the role of volunteers.

8.5 EVALUATING THE RELATIONSHIP WITH THE INFORMAL SECTOR

In the first part of this section we shall discuss divisional managers' assessments and the extent to which they succeeded in mobilising the informal sector of care. In the second part we shall concentrate on the children and the success of the Project in providing each child with a significant relationship outside the Project.

Divisional Managers' Assessments

Divisional managers felt that they had been successful in mobilising some parts of the informal sector. They felt that they had most success in enhancing the relationships between the children and their relatives.

The divisional managers felt that the relatives had responded very well to the opportunities offered by the Project. In no instance had family or parental contact diminished. Indeed there were some notable successes in consolidating relationships between the children and their families. The divisional managers felt that they had most success when they could build on existing relationships. For example, David's parents visited him once a week whilst he was in hospital and took him out for a car ride at weekends. In the Project not only did David's parents visit him but other members of the family, notably his younger sister, started visiting. In addition, they increased their range of activities. His parents became involved in his care and also did odd jobs around the bungalow and helped with other children. The divisional managers accepted that they had been less successful in reconstituting relationships with parents that had atrophied while the children had been in hospital. Generally, parents had withdrawn from the contact with their children in hospital for a reason. For example, there had been tensions in some families about the most appropriate form of care. These complex tensions were difficult to address and the Project staff accepted that in some cases parents chose to maintain low levels of contact with their children.

Generally the divisional managers felt happy about the relationships they had with the other residents on Croxteth Park Estate. Before the Project opened there was some hostility but once it opened there was very little. When a hostile article appeared in one of the local free papers, neighbours actively defended the Project. The project staff and children were able to use the estate and local amenities in just the same way as other households. They had also been able to contribute to the Estate through the Neighbourhood Watch Scheme and by offering help to their neighbours.

The relationship with individual neighbours varied. Phase Two had developed closer contact with its neighbours than Phase One. Phase Two staff at the time of the research had close friendships with two of its neighbours and exchanged support with these two neighbours. One family often visited and went for walks with the staff and the children. A second household became involved. A teenager had developed a close relationship with one of the children, Margaret, and visited the house regularly. In Phase One there was only one such close relationship. One of the neighbours was a domestic worker in the Project and her family visited. When Phase One was short staffed this domestic was recruited as a part-time R.S.W. as she had previous experience of nursery nursing. Her two sons visited Rob.

The divisional managers felt that the differences between the two parts of the Project in their relationships with neighbours could be explained by their location and the time of their move. Phase One had fewer neighbours and Barnardo's moved in after the other residents. In some senses Barnardo's was the late comer. In both phases local children acted as an important point of contact. Young children tended to call and play with the children. In each phase friendships have been established between local children and children in the Project. In Phase Two the parents followed their children. For example, parents have visited to ensure that the R.S.W.s did not mind if their children came to play.

The divisional managers were disappointed with the extent to which they had achieved their objectives for volunteers. Their target was 24 volunteers. From the 60 enquiries to the initial two advertisements they succeeded in recruiting 17 volunteers but two of these volunteers did not start. Only one of the original volunteers continued visiting but she developed a very strong commitment to the Project. She visited three times a week and developed a close relationship with one of the most handicapped children, Mark. She attended his six-monthly review meetings and became his respite foster parent. The other volunteers stopped visiting for a variety of reasons. For the older volunteers ill-health and family crises such as a bereavement tended to be major factors. For younger volunteers transport difficulties tended to be important. The Project was difficult to reach by public transport and many of the volunteers did not have their own transport and lived some distance away.

The divisional managers were generally happy about the development of the Project's relationship with neighbours on the estate but they felt that they may not have made sufficient allowance for the nature of Croxteth Park Estate. It is an area of owner-occupier housing and there is relatively limited interaction between neighbours. When the Project opened, it was a relatively new estate with few developed social networks. The norm was one of respecting privacy. The divisional managers felt that they may have been too positive in announcing the presence of the Project. For example, the initial house-warming party and invitations to the neighbours to visit were not normal features of the estate. If they were setting up a similar Project they would place greater emphasis on moving into their houses as unobtrusively as possible and would want to be treated as four normal households:

> My view is that we should keep a low profile, not "we're Barnardo's, we're here"... We just want to be seen as living there.

Divisional managers were least happy with the process of recruiting and using the volunteers. They accepted it was a mistake to try and start the first group of volunteers at the same time as the first group of staff. The staff needed time to develop confidence and experience in caring for the children. The introduction of the volunteers at the same time was an unnecessary strain. The volunteers expected and wanted to work with the children but the staff did not feel sufficiently confident to allow them to do so. The volunteers should have been introduced later when the staff were established in their roles and had time to supervise the volunteers properly.

Using similar processes to recruit and train staff and volunteers was not a success. They were too formal. As the Project developed, so the process of recruiting volunteers changed. Volunteers were recruited through the social networks of the Project, i.e. either acquaintances of the Project staff, neighbours or former staff who wanted to maintain their contact. Only one of the eight active volunteers at the time of the research had been formally recruited. Four were acquaintances of Project staff, two were former Project staff and one was a neighbour.

When the first volunteers were recruited, the divisional managers saw their role as complementary to the staff. They expected volunteers to befriend specific children. Many of the planning discussions were about the type of activities the volunteers should perform and the amount of contact they should have with children. Tasks tended to be divided into three groups: those that involved close contact with the children such as bathing, those that involved less intimate contact such as playing and those that involved no contact at all such as gardening. The Project staff clearly felt that volunteers should primarily be involved in play-type activities. As the relationship between the volunteers and the Project has developed, so it has become clear that this formal specification of the role of volunteers was not helpful. Some volunteers wanted to develop close relationships with specific children and wanted to be closely involved in their care. However, other volunteers did not want to be involved in this way. They wanted to be useful, e.g. by doing odd jobs. Of the eight volunteers, four developed close relationships with specific to children. Two volunteers played with the children but had no exclusive relationship with a specific child. Two volunteers had minimal contact with the children and did odd jobs, clerical work and gave people lifts. The project staff accepted that it was important to allow volunteers to develop their own activities.

The Children and the Informal Sector

One of the major objectives of the Project was to provide each child with a range of significant relationships outside the Project. In this section we shall discuss each child's social network and the way it has developed in the Project. In the hospitals the children could be grouped into three categories: children who had well-developed and close relationships with their families, David, Barbara and Anne; children who had limited contact with their families but who had developed relationships with other adults, Margaret and Ivan; and children who did not have active relationships outside the hospital, Rob, Linda, Mark and Sean.

David's parents visited him every weekend in hospital and took him out for a car ride. They became very involved in the Project. They visited regularly and not only were they closely involved in David's care but they also helped with other children and did odd jobs. The open house atmosphere of the Project meant that other members of David's family started to visit. In particular David began to develop a relationship with his sister, whom he had rarely seen while he was in hospital.

David was in Phase One and as the neighbours of this phase were more "distant", he had limited interaction with the neighbours and their children. However, David developed a close relationship with Marion, an 18 year old volunteer. She visited David on Thursday evenings and attended his review meetings.

Barbara also had a close relationship with her parents while she was in the hospital and this relationship developed in the same way as David's. Barbara went home every weekend and her parents became involved in the Project. They made friends with the other children in Phase One.

As Barbara lived in Phase One, she had developed little contact with the neighbours and their children. However, Barbara developed close relationships with two volunteers. Tom, a retired local authority joiner, was a friend of the Project leader. He was recruited as a volunteer in the summer of 1984 and he visited Barbara every Monday night. He developed a very close relationship with Barbara, was closely involved in her care and attended her review meetings. Tony was 35 and he was recruited in the same way and at the same time as Tom. He visited every Tuesday evening and he also developed a relationship with

Relatives, Neighbours and Volunteers

Barbara although not quite as close as Tom. He attended her review meetings.

Anne entered Phase Two of the Project in June 1985. Her parents had visited her frequently in hospital and maintained this close relationship when she was transferred. Anne went home every weekend. Although Anne did not develop a close relationship with a volunteer she did develop a friendship with a neighbour, Kay a teenage girl who lived near the Project. Kay had initially developed a close friendship with Margaret. Kay visited nearly every evening.

When *Margaret* was in hospital, her relationship with her parents had atrophied. However, Margaret had developed a close relationship with a family who offered her respite foster care and this relationship was maintained when she was transferred to the Project. The foster parents took her home for weekends. When she was in the Project this relationship was developed and her respite foster parents decided to apply to become her full-time foster parents. In December 1984 Margaret went to live with her foster parents on a full-time basis.

While she was living in the Project, Margaret had no particular friendship with a volunteer. However, she did develop a very close relationship with Kay who visited Margaret most days and invited her to tea. Despite Margaret's severe handicap the Project staff agreed that she could visit and subsequently Margaret visited Kay regularly. Following Margaret's move to her foster parents, Kay maintained contact with her. For example, she visited her in hospital when she was ill.

Ivan, like Margaret, had minimal contact with his parents but had developed a close relationship with a respite foster parent over several years. This relationship was maintained and enhanced when Ivan was admitted to the Project and his respite foster mother continued to take him home at weekends. She decided to apply to become his full-time foster parent and she was accepted by Barnardo's. However, she lived in a one-bedroom local authority flat and she could not take Ivan on a permanent basis until she had been rehoused. There was a long local authority waiting list and both Ivan's respite foster mother and divisional managers had to place considerable pressure on the housing authority before it agreed to rehouse Ivan's respite foster mother. In November 1985 Ivan went to live with her on a full-time basis. Ivan was in Phase Two of the Project and he benefitted from the general higher level of contact that children in this phase had with the neighbours and their children. Although he had no specific friendships, the local children played with him when they visited. Additionally Ivan developed a relationship with Nicola, a volunteer who was in her mid-twenties. She was a R.S.W. until 1985 and she wanted to retain contact with the Project. She visited about once a week and spent time with Ivan.

Mark had occasional contact with his mother while he was in hospital and they maintained the same level of contact after he moved to the Project. In view of this limited relationship, Mark was considered at an early stage for the fostering programme and was one of the first children to move to the full-time care of foster parents.

As Mark was in the second phase, he benefitted from the higher level of interaction with neighbours that was characteristic of this phase. When local children visited they played with him, but he did not have any particular friendship. However, Mark developed a close relationship with a volunteer. Wendy was in her mid-forties and was recruited in the original volunteer recruitment programme in the summer of 1983. She developed and maintained a very close relationship with Mark. While he was in the Project, she visited him every Monday, Thursday and Saturday evenings. She attended his review meetings. Indeed her relationship developed so well with Mark that she applied to become, and was accepted as, his respite foster parent. Following his move to full-time foster parents she has remained as his respite foster parent.

Linda's parents had very little contact with her when she lived in hospital. Until the end of 1983 they lived abroad and therefore could not visit her regularly. They did return to live in England but still lived over 100 miles from Liverpool. They did not visit the Project but maintained contact by telephone. When Linda was ill and had to go into hospital for an eye operation, her parents became more involved and were in regular communication with the Project about her progress. In Linda's case social work support was vital. Linda was a source of some tension within the family. Following discussions with the social worker from the fostering team, they agreed that Linda should have the opportunity of normal family life and that she should be considered for full-time foster placement.

Linda lived in Phase Two of the Project and, although she had no specific friendship with neighbours, she was extremely popular with the neighbours and local children. She had regular visitors.

Linda developed a close relationship with a volunteer, Karen, who was 18 and lived across the road. She visited the Project initially as a neighbour and in May 1985 she applied to be a volunteer. She visited most evenings and spent most of her time with Linda.

The development of *Rob's* relationships were rather similar to those of Linda and showed the benefits of good social work support. When Rob was in hospital his parents appeared to have rejected him. Following his admission, the foster team social worker visited his parents regularly and tried to get them to discuss his future. Initially, they were hostile to Rob and refused to even acknowledge he had a future. For example, they would not even give permission for the use of antibiotics. However, following considerable efforts by the Project staff and field social worker they suddenly agreed that Rob should be fostered. As Rob's parents had come to this difficult decision and in view of the major change in attitudes it represented, divisional managers felt it was important that they should react quickly and positively. They convened a special case conference to discuss Rob's future. This accepted Rob into the fostering scheme and a special arrangement was made to find a foster family for him. A family was identified that already had two young children and the relationship between Rob and his foster family rapidly developed. He was transferred to the care of his foster parents at the beginning of July 1985.

Rob was in Phase One of the Project and, despite the fairly limited interactions with neighbours, Rob succeeded in developing close friendships with the children of one of the neighbours. Maria was a domestic in Phase One and she visited the Project both as a neighbour and as a domestic. A close relationship developed between her sons and Rob. They came to play with Rob regularly. Although Rob did not develop a specific relationship with a volunteer, all three of the original volunteers that visited during the winter of 1983/84 played with him.

When *Sean* was in hospital he had limited contact with his parents. This did not change after he entered the Project. Sean was in Phase One and perhaps suffered from the more limited contact with the informal sector of Phase One. The neighbours were less involved and only three volunteers visited Phase One. Sean had little interaction with the neighbours and volunteers that did visit. Neither did he have respite foster parents. Of all the children, Sean seemed to have benefitted least from the Project's commitment to developing relationships with the informal sector.

It was difficult to explain why Sean did not develop more positive relationships. Part of the problem seemed to stem from Sean's past experience. In hospital, Sean was a fairly withdrawn child who was rather suspicious of strangers. He was a very attractive child but he was not immediately appealing in the same way as Rob or Linda. He also came to live in the Project in November 1984, over a year after it opened. By the time Sean entered many of the relationships with the informal sector were already well established.

Sean's situation did draw attention to some of the limitations of the process of relating to the informal sector of care. The Project staff accepted that they had to allow individuals in the informal sector to choose the type of relationship they wanted to develop. They placed great emphasis on spontaneity. Normal relationships of friendship develop in this way. However, as carers, the staff also had a commitment to ensuring each child got a fair share of the available resources. One of the major resources was the informal sector. It was difficult to balance choice with fairness when some children were more immediately appealing than others. In most cases it would appear that the staff were able to achieve a fair balance. When children did not develop relationships with individuals in one part of the informal sector, the Project staff were able to locate relationships in another. Sean was the only example in which this balancing was unsuccessful.

Comment

The involvement of the informal sector in the Project was both important and difficult to manage. It was important because it is a key aspect of everyday life that people develop relationships outside their households. It is one way in which care in the community is different from care in institutions. However, managing the relationship with the informal sector was intrinsically difficult. Members of the informal sector had no obligations to become involved in the Project. If they chose to become involved they could also choose to withdraw.

Divisional managers always accepted that involving the informal sector would be problematic. They felt that they had had some major successes, in particular with the children's families. However, they also recognised that in other areas they had not fully achieved their objectives. Relationships with neighbours of Phase One were limited and, of the sixteen volunteers initially recruited, only one developed a long-term relationship with the Project. The divisional managers learned a lot in the process of setting up and running the Project. The link workers were a vital part of maintaining contact with the informal sector, especially parents. The support of parents was crucial. The divisional managers clearly recognised the dangers of over-structuring relationships with the informal sector. Their initial approach to both neighbours and volunteers was probably too formal and they later developed more natural methods. From the point of view of the children the programme appeared to be very successful. The children, with the exception of Sean, developed significant relations outside the Project. They had developed relationships with both adults and children that were an important part of their everyday lives.

8.6 CONCLUSION

The Croxteth Park Project was located within the community and looked to the community for support. In some ways the staff in the Project were like parents caring for mentally handicapped children at home and they exploited the same sources of community support. The Project staff sought to encourage and maintain the involvement of the informal sector and saw it as important both for the development of the children and for the operation of the Project. The Project staff could provide information about the Project and encourage involvement, but the choice as to whether these opportunities were exploited depended upon the relatives, the volunteers and the neighbours. For example, some parents chose to interact frequently and provided a lot of support both for their children and for the Project. Others maintained a more formal and distant relationship, coming only when invited to formal occasions such as reviews.

The Project did not choose its neighbours. The bungalows were established in a specific location and Barnardo's had no control over the people who chose to buy houses in the same location. The Project faced something of a dilemma in its relationships with neighbours. The relationships with friends/volunteers was voluntary but interaction with neighbours was a result of having chosen accommodation in the same neighbourhood. The Project shared the neighbourhood with neighbours and yet had a rather different relationship to it. The interaction with neighbours varied. Some neighbours had developed fairly close and intimate relationships with the unit, but most chose to retain a relationship of benign neutrality. They were friendly but did not chose too become too closely involved (see Alaszewski and Chappell, 1987).

Initially the recruitment of volunteers was modelled on the recruitment of staff and similar procedures were used. This was not successful and the overwhelming majority of the initial group of volunteers chose not to maintain it. The subsequent recruitment and relationship of the volunteers was modelled far more on patterns of friendship. Volunteers were recruited through friendship networks and they came to the Project because they enjoyed it. This appeared to provide a far more stable and fruitful basis for the involvement of volunteers.

9 EDUCATION AND HEALTH: CO-ORDINATING SERVICES

ALISON MORRIS AND ANDY ALASZEWSKI

Children with a profound mental handicap cannot live in the community without the support of a network of services. Between them, the statutory and voluntary agencies must supply the comprehensive care previously provided in the long-stay hospital. In this chapter we shall examine the ways in which Barnardo's mobilised statutory services to provide the children in the Project with health and educational services.

9.1 COLLABORATION AND CO-ORDINATION: MANAGING RELATIONS BETWEEN AGENCIES

There is growing recognition that as the magnitude and scope of government activities increase, so the very size and complexity of administrative structures create disorganisation. For example, Faludi has argued that specialisation between agencies

> isolates agents dealing with different aspects of the same problem and thereby results in disjointed attempts at its solutions. (Faludi, 1973, p.209)

In theory there is a general commitment to co-ordinating the activities of agencies such as the NHS and local authority personal social services. As Wildavsky has pointed out co-ordination has become so generally accepted that it is "one of the golden words of our time" (1979). Although service providers generally accept the principle that they "should contribute to a common purpose at the appropriate time and in the right amount to achieve co-ordination" (1979, p.132), in practice co-ordination seems difficult, if not impossible, to achieve. (see for example NAHA, 1985, Wistow and Fuller, 1983 and 1986, and Booth, 1981). Central government has acknowledged that the lack of effective collaboration is an impediment to the development of community care (D.H.S.S., 1981d, para.1.2).

If organisations share the same objectives and operate through similar processes, then co-ordination should be relatively easy. But where organisations differ in their objectives and have different structures and processes then, as Harrison and Tether have pointed out, co-ordination is not collaboration but coercion (1987). In the 1970's and 1980's researchers examining the process of inter-organisational interaction identified several major issues: the differences in participants' objectives, the importance of networks and the role of resources.

Smith and Cantley have argued that participants in an organisation, for example managers, service providers and clients, have their own goals and that these goals may differ (Smith and Cantley, 1985). The objectives of the different participants are related to their differing perceptions. Participants have varying abilities or power to impose their definitions and to achieve their particular objectives.

Glennerster et al. (1983a and 1983b) used this approach to examine collaboration through joint planning between health and personal social services. N.H.S. officers tended to view planning as a technical exercise and relied heavily on national guidelines and national information. Local government officers tended to see planning as competition between different departments for limited and shrinking resources. They generally disregarded national guidelines and used information to support their particular case. Glennerster et al. showed that it was impossible to understand the nature of collaboration without examining the objectives and intentions of the individuals who were expected to collaborate.

A second major research theme concerned the specific patterns of relations or networks between participants in different organisations. For some participants, their relationship with individuals in other organisations is as important, if not more important, than their relationships in their own organisation. Friend et al. (1974) referred to these individuals as reticulists who could use their social networks to co-ordinate the activities of different organisations.

McKeganey and Hunter (1986) used this approach to examine

Education and Health

the co-ordination of services for elderly people in one area of Scotland. A team of four doctors co-ordinated the activities of the N.H.S. and local authority services by negotiating patient exchanges. In its reticulist role the team acted as an arbiter between the two services. For this role the team members had to appear to be neutral and their success depended on the fact that they had no organisational base and no particular axe to grind.

McKeganey and Hunter drew attention to another major variable in inter-organisational relationships: the role of resources and power relations. They argued that the team had a special relationship with the social work department. The team could, and did, act on behalf of the social work department. They had the clinical expertise to negotiate as equals with hospital consultants and they had the skills to carry out independent assessments. McKeganey and Hunter argued that this power dependency relationship with the social work department was essential for the success of the team. It gave them a basis on which to build coalitions. This concern with power and resources as a determinant of inter-organisational relations has been developed by Benson (1975, see also Hall et al., 1977).

Developing Co-ordinated Services for People with a Mental Handicap

When the majority of mentally handicapped people were institutionalised, there was little pressure on the welfare agencies in the community to provide services. The institutions provided for the health, social and, to a limited extent, educational needs of its residents. The development of community care has meant that these services must now be provided in the community:

> Community care for the mentally handicapped means an alternative to life in large hospitals. It means that they are able to participate in community life and make use of the same range of medical and social services which are available to the main stream of society, and that they visit hospitals as day or out-patients rather than reside in them. But more than this, community care refers to a range of services provided by the employment, education and social services departments of local authorities. (Donges, 1982)

By the 1980s it was generally accepted that, whilst the ideal would be for every mentally handicapped child to remain with his or her family, the most suitable alternative was to provide a life in the community as close as possible to that of "ordinary" family life (Towell, 1980). To achieve this, small residential units would be established, serving the local population. The King's Fund working group stressed that such units would have to be integrated with other local services:

> No residential service can stand alone. It must be closely integrated with other day-to-day services and with those which provide occasional but still essential help. (Towell, 1980, p.19)

Such integration is essential for children with severe mental and physical handicaps. Wessex R.H.A. has established Locally Based Hospital Units for mentally handicapped children, one of which, the Old Rectory, takes only those with a severe enough handicap to be defined as a "health service responsibility". The Unit staff can only manage to care for severely handicapped children because they receive support from professionals in other fields, the local G.P., two paediatricians, the senior nursing officer, clinical psychologist, a psychiatrist and the local special school (Shearer, 1981, p.38).

In Ashington, Northumberland Health Authority has opened three houses for children from Northgate Hospital. The Authority pledged in 1981 to move out fifteen children who still lived in a hospital ward. Support services were provided by the local G.P. and health visitor, community nursing officer, psychologists and social worker (based at the hospital). Unfortunately the children had to return to Northgate for schooling, but ideally they should attend the local special school (Shearer, 1981, p.36) and obviously the co-operation of the local education authority in this matter would be very important.

Both examples emphasise the importance of inter-professional collaboration when residential units are established by health authorities. If the residential service is provided by a local authority or a voluntary agency, the process becomes even more complex and collaboration at the planning level is also essential.

For voluntary agencies providing residential care collaboration is exceedingly important. The MENCAP Homes Foundation specialises in placing adults in ordinary houses, but faces the same problems as projects dealing with children:

Education and Health

> Close co-operation between MENCAP, local councils and health authorities in establishing and running the homes is vital. (MENCAP, 1985)

To achieve this the charity has established Area Management Committees, with representatives from each of these authorities, for each group of homes.

Comment

These examples of community care initiatives illustrate the necessity for inter-agency collaboration and joint working at practitioner level. None of the projects could provide comprehensive care for severely handicapped children without the support of the health, education and social services departments whose professionals provide locally based support.

9.2 CO-OPERATION OR CONFLICT? THE CONGRUENCE OF OBJECTIVES

Barnardo's Objectives

Within the Division, all the staff shared a commitment to the development of the children. However, different staff groups related to the children in different ways. Divisional managers were responsible for obtaining the resources for the children's care and for monitoring the progress of the children. The care staff provided the day-to-day care.

The status of the Project as an experimental unit placed divisional managers in a difficult position. On the one hand they wanted to demonstrate that they could provide a better quality service and on the other hand they required the co-operation of these agencies to provide a comprehensive package of care for the children. The divisional managers wanted to provide care through

> the use of means which are valued in our Society in order to develop and support personal behaviour experiences and characteristics which are likewise valued. (O'Brien and Tyne, 1981)

Their aim was to move children out of long-stay hospitals because they felt such hospitals could not provide this sort of care. However, they did not want the Croxteth Park Project to be a mini-institution providing total 24 hour care, and therefore they felt it was important to use the local health and education services. The divisional managers recognised the importance of services provided by other agencies and felt that each child needed his or her own network of support services. The Project Leader argued that

> Any group of professionals... who can offer something that will enhance the life of any, or all, of the children (are important). That ranges from psychologists, through to teachers, speech therapists, physiotherapists, social workers - you can't put limits on it because it depends very much on the individual needs of the children... If there is a lack of co-operation, if there is a shortfall in terms of the quality of service, in any of the areas, the kids are going to suffer. Now it doesn't mean the Unit will grind to a halt ... but it will reduce the quality of life for the children and their opportunity to develop.

The divisional managers recognised that they had to have well-established links with health care practitioners. The children's high levels of dependency and past medical histories meant that minor health problems could rapidly develop into life-threatening illnesses. The Project leader described one child in the following way:

> Take Mark as an example ... he has got a virtually permanent health problem with the infection trapped in his lung - so physiotherapy is very important for him. He can contract a severe chest condition very quickly. So we've got to be able to pick up those links, they've got to be established.

The involvement of health practitioners was important but tended to be episodic. The school teachers took over responsibility for the children's care during school-time. Therefore continuity of care depended on effective communication between Project staff and teachers. The divisional managers expected teachers to be involved in achieving the objectives of each child's long-term goal plan, although they accepted that it might be difficult to communicate the objectives of the short-term plans.

The divisional managers were not only concerned with ensuring that statutory agencies provided the necessary support in the short term. They were also concerned about the longer-term provision of resources. The D.H.S.S. had agreed to provide the majority of the funds for the eight places in the Project for a minimum of three years and a maximum of 6 years. They had not agreed to fund the foster placements. Therefore the divisional managers had to find the resources for the foster placements and to fund the Project after 6 years.

Barnardo's care staff had day-to-day responsibility for the provision of the care. They needed the help and co-operation of professionals in other agencies to provide comprehensive care. The children's care was structured through a therapeutic programme of developmental and goal plans. To implement these plans the R.S.W.s needed the advice and support of specialists, such as psychologists, speech therapists and physiotherapists, and the co-operation of the school teachers who would provide some of the children's care.

As the care staff were committed to the principles of normalisation, they were concerned not only with the development of the children, but also with ensuring that the care children received indicated that they were socially valued people. These concerns could be seen in the concept of age-appropriateness. The care staff believed that the children should be dressed in a way that was appropriate for their chronological age. For example, a teenage child, who was doubly incontinent, should wear jeans rather than track suit trousers. The jeans were age appropriate, although the track suit trousers were easier to change when wet. When the children attended school the R.S.W.s had to persuade school staff to dress them in age-appropriate clothes. This conflicted with the school teachers' views that comfort and convenience should be of primary importance.

Resources

All the professionals interviewed expressed a commitment to the principles of collaboration, but there were two major impediments; resources and attitudes. The resource implications of the Project varied between the three main statutory agencies, social services, education and health services.

For *Social Services*, especially in Liverpool, the Project was a potential drain on resources. When the children were in hospital, they made very little use of social services resources, however there was a danger for social services that they might be expected to fund the foster placements. The social services were willing to co-operate with Barnardo's as long as it did not commit any of their hard-pressed resources.

Education The children's move from hospital to the Croxteth Park Project did not alter the L.E.A.'s legal responsibilities and therefore had marginal resource implications. In initial contacts, the divisional managers were assured that the L.E.A. would provide the necessary resources for the children's education.

There were some ways in which the Project could make demands on L.E.A. resources. If the divisional managers did not feel that the current placements were suitable then they might request a statement of a child's educational needs. The statement procedure makes demands on limited resources, particularly educational psychologists, and the statement might indicate that a child should receive a different, and possibly more expensive, education.

Barnardo's, as a voluntary agency, was also in a good position to act as an advocate for the children and in this way exert greater pressure for educational resources than parents. For example, Barnardo's held six- monthly review meetings and invited school teachers to attend. One deputy head described the resource implications in the following way:

> I wish that the children (6 attended this school) were physically nearer because they're on the other side of Liverpool and it seems quite a distance to get people to case conferences... from our point of view it's a big hassle.

However at another school, the teachers minimised these resource implications.

Liverpool Health Authority had a commitment to the closure of large long-stay mental handicap hospitals and the Croxteth Park Project was an important means of achieving that objective. Furthermore for a period of between three and six years, the Project was a "free resource". The Health Authority was willing to provide resources for the Project, although not from their main budget. For example, the Authority was willing to use earmarked monies to fund the foster care of the children and to support the longer-term development of the Project.

When the children were in hospital, the medical and

paramedical services were all funded by the hospital budget. When the children moved to the Project many of these services had to be funded by the Family Practitioner Committee or the community services budget. As the Family Practitioner Committee budget was not cash-limited and the children represented only a small additional responsibility, there was no particular issue for the Family Practitioner Committee. However for community services the resource implications were greater. The children made high demands on very restricted and specialist community resources, especially physiotherapy and speech therapy. Barnardo's recognised in the initial application that this might create a serious problem and suggested that they might have to "buy in" some of these services. The community speech therapist confirmed that her input to the Project was limited by scarce resources:

> I've got such a vast case load that it isn't really possible to be very involved with any particular children or adults that I see, whether or not they're in the unit.

Attitudes

Whereas resources were an organisational issue, attitudes were held by individuals and varied between individuals. Most of the professionals we talked to had positive attitudes towards the work of Barnardo's. They seemed not only to understand, but also to accept, Barnardo's philosophy of normalisation. For example, one health authority planning officer expressed his support for the Project in the following way:

> I liked what I saw, I liked Barnardo's as an organisation. I felt that the set-up was good. I didn't have any alarm bells ringing. You know you can go round some places and think "Oh, my God, not here". I felt it was well monitored and yet homely. There was no sign outside saying "Barnardo's Intensive Support Unit". It just looks like an ordinary bungalow. You just go and ring the door bell, no special thing. Its part of the community... There's no "keep away from us" attitude.

Some professionals admitted that they had originally been sceptical, even hostile, to the Project and its normalisation philosophy. For example, the community dentist felt that working with Barnardo's had altered his attitudes:

> There's a whole philosophy towards care for mentally handicapped people that really hadn't occurred to me until I spoke to them - I think the whole point of view of treating them as individuals really even when they are profoundly mentally handicapped... Sometimes I wonder whether I was never aware of the feedback from these kids because I wasn't looking for it, because I didn't think there was going to be any. When you talk to the staff... you begin to think, well, maybe they are individuals - you pick up what they are giving out - what they're giving out is only small and, if you're not looking for it and you're not open to it, you're going to miss it completely.

Only one group of professionals did not accept, or were critical of, the normalisation philosophy of the Project: the teachers in one special school. This school was located in the grounds of a mental handicap hospital and some of the Project children had attended the school when they lived in the hospital. The teachers did not accept the normalisation philosophy. They felt that the R.S.W.s were inexperienced and unrealistic and that the R.S.W.s devalued the school staff's experience and methods of working. One senior teacher expressed her attitude to the Project in the following way:

> The majority of staff, who've worked with the children here, have worked with them quite a while and they've had quite a lot of experience in dealing with these children over a long period of time. We are realistic in our approach to the work, what we think we can do with the children. That doesn't mean we don't look at the potential in the children, but at the Project some people, particularly the link workers, have aims which are a little unrealistic.

Comment

There were two major impediments to the effective provision of support, resources and attitudes. The resource situation was variable. Some resources, such as educational services and hospital care, were available in the quantity the Project staff required, if not always the quality. Other resources, especially specialist community health services such as physiotherapy and speech therapy, were in short supply.

Even where resources were plentiful, negative attitudes could act as a serious impediment to the co-ordination of services. The Project staff had developed a very clear and positive philosophy towards care. Generally staff in other agencies seemed to accept this philosophy even if, at first, they did not understand its full implications. However, professionals who had long experience of working with children with a mental handicap and who had developed a different philosophy, could interpret the normalisation philosophy as a criticism of their style of work. These professionals tended to see co-ordination as a form of coercion.

9.3 ESTABLISHING WORKING LINKS WITH PROFESSIONALS IN OTHER AGENCIES

The Project Leader: A Networker

The inter-organisational network was centred on Barnardo's and the key figure within the agency was the Project leader. He played an active part in the formation of a network of relations but once this network was established he only intervened when there were problems, e.g. shortages of resources or signs of tension.

Establishing Relations Generally the Project leader did not use formal channels of communication. Instead he used his local knowledge and experience to identify and approach professionals whom he knew had a special interest in providing the type of care he wanted. The Project leader took special care to identify and win the support of key personnel in other agencies. The paediatrician at the Children's Hospital was an influential person in the child care services in Liverpool. The Project leader took special care to keep him informed and involve him in key decisions concerning the children. As we have shown in Chapter 2, Barnardo's was willing to make important concessions for the paediatrician in the selection of the children. As a result, the paediatrician felt that he worked "in partnership" with Project staff over the selection of the children and he used his influence to encourage nurses to work with R.S.W.s.

When he was building up the network of professional support, the Project leader placed great emphasis on personal contact. For example, when he was building up relations with the teachers in the special schools, he did not prepare a formal "fact sheet" about the Project. Instead he visited the school and talked to the teachers about the Project and invited them for coffee at the Project so that they could see for themselves.

Providing Resources Although the statutory agencies had a legal duty to provide services, some services, especially physiotherapy and speech therapy, were just not available. When the children were in hospital they had received a physiotherapy service funded from the hospital budget. When they were transferred to the Project this service was radically curtailed. For two years the Project leader attempted to improve the service by negotiating with the community services and developing various informal arrangements. However, during one review the paediatrician suggested that the children's progress was being retarded because of inadequate physiotherapy. The Project leader decided to use the Project "medical supplies" budget to "buy in" sessional services. A physiotherapist was given a contract to provide two hours of physiotherapy a week.

The concern with resources led the Project leader and the divisional director into protracted negotiations with the head of Planning and Performance Review in Liverpool Health Authority. In 1983 Liverpool Health Authority submitted a bid to Mersey Regional Health Authority for funds to close a large mental handicap hospital in Liverpool. Part of this scheme involved the use of the Croxteth Park Project. The Health Authority was willing to fund foster placements if Barnardo's took "replacement" children from the local hospital. The Project leader and divisional director had a series of meetings with the Head of Planning and Performance Review about the transfer of patients. These meetings culminated in a major joint planning meeting held in April 1986. This meeting was called by the D.H.S.S. to discuss the funding of the Project when the D.H.S.S. funding ceased in 1989. Barnardo's were able to obtain a commitment from the Health Authority to the long-term funding of the Project as a sub-regional resource.

Trouble-shooting In areas of tension, the Project leader used formal methods of collaboration to try to resolve the problems. For example, in one special school in which the staff were not sympathetic to the aims of the Project, he established a monthly meeting with the deputy headmistress so that they could have "frank discussions" of school/Project problems. The meetings did not have set agendas. The Project leader asked Project staff to tell him about any issues that had arisen. He then compiled a set of issues for discussion. Most of these items were information about the Project, e.g. staff changes or progress in the fostering of a child, rather than problems.

The Link Workers

The link workers had to use and maintain the networks of professional support established by the Project leader. They did this by maintaining regular face-to-face contact, establishing, where necessary, more formal methods of transferring information and, in some cases, through joint- working.

Maintaining Regular Contact Like the Project leader, the link workers placed great emphasis on informal face-to-face contact. This could be most clearly seen in the Project's relationship with the school. When the children went to school they were always accompanied by Project staff, and the link workers tried to accompany their child as frequently as possible. At the school the Project staff talked to the children's teachers. For example, one teacher we talked to stated that the link worker took this opportunity to request specific treatments or activities for the children such as leg exercises. Link workers also visited the school during the day and spent time in the classroom. For example when Anne first moved to the Project, her teacher found she was difficult to feed. Anne's link worker visited the school and showed them how Anne was fed at the Project. The school teachers had a general invitation to visit the Project and were specifically invited to social occasions in the Project such as the children's birthday parties and barbeques.

An important aspect of maintaining positive relations was indicating that the contribution of other professionals was important and valued and that their advice was useful. This positive evaluation was very important in maintaining the input from professionals such as the dentist and speech therapist. Following persistent requests from the Project leader, the speech therapist agreed to visit the Project. She did not have the time to provide therapy but advised the link workers on ways of developing the children's feeding and communication skills. Because the staff listened to, and carried out her advice, she felt her visits, although infrequent, were important to the children's development and she maintained them.

Formal Mechanisms In Chapter 6 we showed that the process of planning each child's care involved formal mechanisms for sharing information and making decisions, e.g. in the selection and transfer process and in the six-monthly reviews. Barnardo's also saw the selection and transfer as a collaborative exercise involving ward nurses, medical specialists, hospital specialists, Barnardo's psychologists and care staff and the children's parents. Barnardo's convened a series of joint planning meetings to decide about a child's suitability for placement in the Project and to decide how and when the transfer was to take place. To indicate that they valued the ward staff's contribution to the children's care, the Project staff were willing to compromise one aspect of the normalisation philosophy. The Project staff saw the bungalows as the children's homes and they discouraged "official" visitors. However to encourage ward staff to maintain a relationship with the children Barnardo's offered them an "open invitation" to visit the Project as "friends" of the children whenever they wished. (For a more detailed discussion see Ong and Alaszewski, 1988.)

In addition to the formal meetings, the Project staff utilised "Home-School" diaries to facilitate the flow of information between the Project and the Schools. This diary recorded the significant events that had affected each child and contained questions and queries about problems that were arising or issues that affected the child's welfare at school or in the Project. Any person involved in a child's care could write comments in the diary.

Joint working In some situations collaboration went beyond joint planning or sharing of information to joint working, i.e. staff from the Project worked with and alongside other professionals. This joint working took place mainly in the hospitals, either when a child was being transferred to the Project or when a child was undergoing in-patient treatment.

When Linda was admitted to a local general hospital for surgery, the staff in the surgical ward had no previous experience of working with such a handicapped child. It was agreed that Linda should have a side room, that Project staff would provide Linda's basic care and the ward staff would provide Linda's specialist care and would visit every few hours to check everything was all right. This proved to be a mutually beneficial arrangement. The ward staff could concentrate on Linda's specialist treatment and the Project staff could maintain contact with Linda and make

Education and Health

sure that she was receiving her normal care and treatment. The Project staff were also able to get immediate information about Linda's treatment and training in any procedures which they would need to carry out when Linda returned to the Project.

Comment

The staff in the Project were responsible for maintaining effective networks of professional support. Generally the Project leader established the links and contacts and the link workers maintained the contacts. The Project leader was only involved in areas that were particularly problematic as in relations with the teachers in the special school.

Generally the Project staff felt it was best to use informal methods of establishing and maintaining contact. They laid great stress on developing personal face-to-face contact and only used more structured formal methods such as joint meetings or Home-School diaries where there were specific problems that more informal methods could not cope with.

9.4 ASSESSING THE DEVELOPMENT OF WORKING LINKS

Barnardo's Assessment

Generally the divisional managers believed they had got the process right and felt that there was little need to adjust it. They thought that the informal person-to-person approach created the best way of sharing information and working together.

The managers were generally satisfied with the outcome of collaboration and they felt that professionals in other agencies had responded well and provided a high-quality service. Many community-based residential units have experienced problems with general medical services but the Project leader felt that the Project staff and the G.P. had established "a very good working relationship". The G.P. clearly understood the principles of normalisation and the developmental objectives of the Project. Barnardo's was particularly pleased with the relationship the Project had developed with the local paediatrician. The Project leader felt that the paediatrician commanded the respect of his colleagues and parents and that his positive evaluation of the

Education and Health

Project had been vital in maintaining good working relations between Project staff and the hospital staff.

The care staff in the Project were less concerned with the long-term and "behind-the-scenes" aspects of collaboration and were more concerned with the immediate day-to-day care of the children. They were more conscious of the occasional hiccups in collaboration that tended to occur even when the process generally seemed to work well and professionals in other agencies seemed willing and able to provide the right sort of services. For example, although the community dentist was seen as very helpful, the R.S.W.s sometimes found it difficult to understand the reasons for some of his actions. During a hepatitis scare, the dentist was worried about the risk to the children and refused to see them in the clinic. The R.S.W.s felt that the children were being deprived of a service as they did not understand the dentist's reasons for temporarily suspending the service. Similarly the care staff were disappointed with the response of nurses in the mental handicap hospital to their attempt to maintain relationships with the children. Although the ward nurses visited the Project before the children were transferred, none maintained contact afterwards.

Divisional managers did recognise that there were areas in which collaboration was not successful but they felt that problems were caused either by lack of resources or negative attitudes. The Project leader accepted that Barnardo's faced major problems in establishing effective working relations with physiotherapists and speech therapists. Individual therapists were keen to provide a service but they just did not have the time.

At the time of the research, the speech therapy service for the children was minimal. The physiotherapy service was better. The children received a regular service from a therapist who was committed to the philosophy of the Project and was keen to develop new forms of therapy, such as horse riding. However this service had only been established after two years of relatively fruitless negotiation and divisional managers were very unhappy that they had been forced to make good the inadequacies of the local services by "buying in".

Divisional managers felt that differences in attitudes created a serious impediment to effective collaboration with the teachers in one special school. They were unhappy about the general principle of segregated special education and especially that one of the special schools was located in the grounds of, and associated with a mental handicap hospital. However, given the policy of the education authority, they had to accept this form of education. They were more concerned with the quality of education and care provided in this school.

This concern was shared by the care staff. The care staff felt that the teachers and care staff in the school had very different perceptions of the children. One member of the Project staff described the attitudes of the school staff in the following way:

> The teachers and care assistants tend to see the children as "babies" and tend to see us as staff of a residential unit not as substitute parents. They think of the children as "ill" and send them home when the slightest problem develops. Once they phoned up and said Barbara was dying. We went straight to the school and when we got there she was fine. They tend to talk over the children's heads. One of our staff heard a care worker remark about Anne, in her presence, "she does nothing but shit all day". We made a formal complaint about that.

The Project staff felt that the teachers tended to overemphasise the children's disabilities and ill-health and that they tended to over-react to minor health problems. For example, the school staff seemed unwilling to accept that they could manage Barbara's epilepsy and Anne's asthma. The care staff felt that the Home-School diary should not be used as a sort of nursing or medical record. For example, a link worker successfully argued that it was inappropriate to record his child's bowel actions in the diary.

The Project staff did accept that they might have contributed to some of the friction, especially in the first year when they might not always have been very diplomatic and they might have been rather "over-enthusiastic". The initial training programme for the staff had given them high expectations but had provided them with very little information about the schools and school practices.

Comment Generally the Project staff felt happy with the support and co-operation which they received from professionals in other agencies. Where there were problems, they felt these were caused by scarce resources or negative attitudes. The divisional managers were concerned with the quantity of some of the services they received, especially speech therapy and physiotherapy. For the care staff, it was the day-to-day quality of the service and the relationships that created more concern.

Education and Health

The Views of Other Professionals

Health service professionals were generally impressed with the Project and with the process and outcome of working with Barnardo's. The health professionals welcomed the emphasis Barnardo's placed on developing informal relations. They found it especially helpful in planning major transitions for the children which required careful preparation and could be emotionally demanding, such as the transition from hospital to the Project and the transition from the Project to foster-care. Problems only developed when a third party was involved. For example, when Jennifer was admitted to the Project, two separate education authorities were involved in planning her education. Messages between these two authorities were lost and when Jennifer was admitted to the Project, neither authority had prepared a statement of her educational needs.

Health professionals also found the more formal elements of collaboration helpful, especially the children's reviews. The health professionals who attended found that their contributions were valued and that there was a genuine sharing of information. The only problem was that a relatively narrow group of health service professionals were invited. For example, in the original proposals for the Project the divisional managers stated that they would invite the children's general medical practitioner to attend. When we interviewed the G.P. he told us that he was disappointed that he had not been invited.

Health professionals generally found it easy to work with both the Project leader and the care staff. Several practitioners spoke with great respect about the enthusiasm of the Project leader and the positive way in which he had initiated contact and encouraged their involvement. For example, the dentist had involved his dental health educator in the Project because he felt that "Barnardo's have always been keen for any input available". The paediatrician felt that the Project leader was "instrumental" in establishing a network of collaboration and was the pivotal point in that network.

The R.S.W.s reinforced the positive impression made by the Project leader. Health professionals felt that they valued their expertise and advice. For example, the speech therapist said that the R.S.W.s' commitment to the children made her feel that her visits were worthwhile, even if they were limited in number. The G.P. noted the R.S.W.s' "exemplary" devotion to the children.

Education and Health

Initially health professionals, such as the paediatrician, were cautious about Barnardo's approach. They were not sure whether it would work. However when they saw the improvements in the children, their caution generally changed to enthusiasm. Some professionals said they had learnt from the Project's approach.

Nurses, who had cared for the children in mental handicap hospitals, had less positive views of collaboration. As we showed in Chapter 3, they had very negative views about the process of selecting and transferring the first eight children. They felt that Barnardo's had improved the process and ward nurses were now genuinely involved in and shared the decision-making. One ward sister commented that she had visited the Project and had seen the improvement in the children and their quality of life. She and other nurses now had more faith in Barnardo's and its staff. However, ward nurses still had some reservations about the Project. One nurse described her feelings about the transfer of one child in the following way:

> The Barnardo's people think that they can do better than we do, and they made us feel that we didn't do enough for her.

Some nurses felt that Barnardo's staff were insensitive and over-powering on the day they took over responsibility and they felt that the child was being taken from them.

Relations between the Project and staff in the schools varied. At most schools the staff were very positive about Barnardo's. However at one special school the teachers did not feel that effective collaboration took place. In view of the problems at this school we shall concentrate on it.

Teachers, at this school, identified a problem in the process of collaboration. They did not feel that the objectives and working principles of the Project had been fully explained to them when the Project opened. In particular, they felt that two issues fundamental to the working of the Project, normalisation and fostering, were not adequately explained:

> Looking back, we had to work it out for ourselves; a lot of people were baffled.

The teachers did not feel that they had received adequate information about the purpose of the Project. In particular they did not receive information about the fostering programme. They felt that this communication problem had caused a degree of resentment and "disillusionment" among some members of the school staff, who had believed the Project would provide the children with "a home forever". One teacher described the Project as "a clearing house for fostering".

The staff at this school did not believe that Barnardo's valued their contribution to caring for the children. The school staff felt that Barnardo's acted in a "high-handed" manner at the time, and the Head Teacher stated that the school still found the agency staff "over-powering", because of the high level of their enthusiasm.

The school staff had very different responsibilities from those of the Project staff. The teachers worked with a number of children and could not develop a close one-to-one relationship with each child. They wanted to stimulate each child but as they were dealing with large numbers of children, they had to provide this stimulation within the framework of a clear routine of daily activities. The school staff believed that Barnardo's did not value this approach and that Barnardo's staff were more interested in using unusual activities, such as computer education, to stimulate the children. The school staff felt that they were in competition with the Project staff. One teacher described this in the following way:

> It irritates me in a way, we haven't much time in school, we can't spend all day with one particular child but yes, we would like to know what the goal plans were.

At the time of the research the school staff had little understanding of the role they were expected to take in working with Barnardo's. Two teachers felt that the only reason for the children attending school was to meet the normalisation objective. They argued that it seemed a pointless expense for Barnardo's to send the children to school when the Project had its own psychologist and physiotherapist devising goal plans and programmes. The major feeling was one of redundancy. The school staff did not feel involved in the children's education when they could see that the Project had all the necessary resources and had chosen not to involve them in goal planning. The feelings were also evident in discussions of the six-monthly reviews, in which teachers expressed their disappointment that the role of the school could be dealt with in three or four lines of a report. This was based on a misunderstanding as divisional managers expected teachers to contribute their own "school" report and felt that they would be eroding the role of the teachers if they wrote a longer section on the children's education.

The school staff felt that Barnardo's approach was "unrealistic" and that normalisation, for some children, was being taken too far. For example, the teacher and care assistant both stated that the children's clothes were unsuitable. The teachers felt that the practical care needs should be given precedence over abstract principles, e.g. that for any child who was incontinent or non-ambulant soft tracksuit bottoms would be both more normal and more comfortable attire. The appearance of a child should be of secondary consideration to comfort and convenience.

School staff accepted that the co-ordination of work between the school and the Project was not as effective as it could be. They felt that collaboration designed to promote effective joint working such as reviews, Home-School diary, Project Leader/Deputy Head Teacher meetings and informal Link Worker-Teacher contact, had been only partially successful. For example, the Deputy Head commented that reviews could be "quite useful" if issues were followed up, but could become "horrendous" affairs when "them and us" situations developed.

Despite these problems, the school staff acknowledged that the Project had been successful in many ways. Anne's and David's teacher said:

> They are a hundred times better for being in the unit, health wise and in happiness. There is no question that their lives have been changed by being in the unit.

The potential for a good working relationship between the school and Project staff existed but had not been exploited. With only one exception the staff at the school expressed a belief that at a personal level the working relationship was reasonably good. The problems seem to relate not to personalities but to a lack of information on and understanding of the Project's aims and working methods. The ineffectiveness of communication about these issues was an impediment to effective collaboration.

9.5 SUMMARY AND COMMENT

If community-based residential units are to provide high-quality care for children with a profound mental handicap, then it is vital that they develop a network of support and mobilise the commitment and enthusiasm of professionals in other agencies. If the staff in a project fail to mobilise this support then either the health and development of the children will suffer or else the Project will become a "mini-institution" reproducing the comprehensive care provided within the hospitals.

Barnardo's were concerned about both the quality and quantity of support services. They did not want their children to receive the bare minimum. They wanted their children to have a high-quality service that enabled them to develop their potential and indicated that they were valued people.

As far as possible Barnardo's relied on informal methods to develop and maintain the network of support. Formal methods were occasionally required but used by themselves would only result in the provision of a minimum service. The Project leader played a key role in identifying professionals who were sympathetic to the style and objective of the Project and developing a relationship with them. Once he had established this relationship, he trusted his staff to maintain it and only become involved when there were specific areas of tension.

Generally this approach worked very well. The children received the health care and education they required and Barnardo's established a network of supportive professionals. There were only two impediments, resources and attitudes. In some cases, the necessary support services did not exist, e.g. physiotherapy and speech therapy. In this situation the Project could use some of its own resources to "buy in" a service. However, the protracted negotiations involved meant that for a time the children did not receive the high-quality physiotherapy and speech therapy which Barnardo's wanted.

Attitudes could be more of an impediment. Paradoxically, Barnardo's found it easier to work with professionals who had limited experience of children with profound mental handicap. Professionals with limited experience generally had no established work patterns and had no clear view of the best way of providing care or therapy. Thus the staff in Croxteth Park Project found it relatively easy to persuade these professionals of the benefits of the normalisation approach. Staff with extensive experience had established ways of caring for these children and had their own philosophy of care, albeit this philosophy was frequently implicit. Project staff found it more difficult to persuade these professionals to change their approach.

10 THE PSYCHOLOGICAL DEVELOPMENT OF THE CHILDREN

STEVEN LOVETT

In this chapter I shall describe the psychological development of those children selected for the Croxteth Park Project. In the first section I shall discuss the methods which I used to assess the children. In the second section I will illustrate the type of developmental changes that have been found by describing the development of three children.

10.1 ASSESSING CHILDREN WITH A PROFOUND MENTAL HANDICAP

As the Croxteth Park Project was an experimental unit, it was important that Barnardo's had a clear and precise set of criteria for assessing the suitability of the children for admission to the Project. In the original application to the D.H.S.S., Barnardo's had a loose definition of the term "profound and multiple mental handicap". As a psychologist, I felt it was important to provide a precise definition. Traditional definitions are both imprecise and rather negative. For example, traditionally profound mental handicap has often been defined as a performance on an IQ test of less than 20 or an "untestable" result. This type of result would not be related to a child's chronological age or physical handicap. This type of definition is so crude that it is virtually meaningless. Instead I adopted Landesman-Dwyer's (1974) developmental and behavioural definition of profound and multiple mental handicap as

* an extreme limited responsiveness to external stimulation
* an obvious severe neuro-muscular dysfunction;

The Psychological Development of the Children

* an inability to move through space by any means other than simple turning;
* an inability to achieve or maintain a seated position; poor head control;
* the existence of records indicating "hopeless" prognosis for behaviour and physiological development, even with treatment.

In developmental terms such profoundly and multiply mentally handicapped children should not manifest behaviour more advanced than that would be expected from a six-month old infant.

Clarke and Clarke (1984) suggest that assessment has four main functions. These are:

* To describe the individual as he or she is at a particular point in time, in terms of intellectual, social, emotional, educational or other characteristics so that the individual can be compared with a normative or contrast group of individuals;
* To predict the individual's intellectual, social, emotional, educational or other characteristics at later points in time;
* To provide a profile of an individual's behavioural assets and deficits as a starting point for remedial programmes;
* To provide a base line against which the personal or social development of an individual or group can be assessed.

Kiernan and Jones (1977) identify a similar range of possible functions:

* *Administratively Oriented Assessment* The purpose of this type of testing is administrative and aims to place an individual in an appropriate service;
* *Criterion Referenced Assessment* The purpose of this type of testing is to correctly place the individual in an educational programme and as such would reflect the curriculum objectives appropriate for the group;
* *Functional Analysis or Micro-Assessment* The purpose of this type of assessment is to directly modify specific responses within a given individual. Here assessment and intervention are interrelated processes.

It is important that assessment procedures are related to the objectives of the assessment. In this study there were two major objectives. To assess the appropriateness of the children's admission to the Project and to demonstrate the ways in which the children responded to their new environment. In order to achieve this, I used several different assessment tests to give as detailed a profile of changes in skill levels as possible.

Problems in Using Standardised Tests

Hogg and Mittler (1980) suggest that the psychological assessment of mentally handicapped people is important as it is the cornerstone of effective intervention. Unfortunately few assessment instruments exist which can be used with severely and profoundly mentally handicapped people. These people suffer from additional disabilities such as physical handicap and sensory impairment, which seriously affect their ability to perform appropriately on standardised assessment tests. Such additional disabilities have been shown to increase proportionally with degrees of mental handicap (Hutton, Talkington and Altman, 1973). Thus, Berkson and Landesman-Dwyer (1977) conclude that many individuals are classified as profoundly mentally handicapped simply because they cannot be assessed using existing procedures.

The use of standardised assessment tests with severely and profoundly mentally handicapped people has been seriously questioned over a number of years (Baumeister, 1965; Ross and Boroskin, 1972). Although their overall usefulness is limited, they do have some predictive validity even at the very low end of the intellectual distribution (Berkson and Landesman-Dwyer, 1977). Shakespeare (1970) shows that standardised intelligence tests have some value with individuals who perform at a developmental age of over 18 months but that their usefulness rapidly declines with increasing handicap.

Some common problems identified by psychologists when using existing assessment procedures with the most handicapped children include: the tests' lack of standardisation at lower levels of functioning; that performance on these tests is only a limited and partial description of behaviour; that IQ is no guide for treatment intervention; and that standardised tests cannot be applied in a standardised manner. The experimental work of many British psychologists in the late 1950s and early 1960s has shown that severely and profoundly mentally handicapped people's performance on their first trial of an item is not a good indicator of their subsequent performance. Intelligence tests which present items on a one-trial basis have little value with severely and profoundly mentally handicapped people. However, as Berger and Yule (1985) have indicated, repeat testing may be of benefit in investigating deterioration in such individuals.

Hogg and Mittler (1980) argue that different tests use different models to explain and predict the development of behaviour. There are three main models:

* Skill-Oriented
* Piagetian
* Radical behaviourist.

The three models of behavioural development are based on different theories of human growth and development and are related to different methods of assessing this.

Psychologists, using the skill-oriented model, see behaviour as a repertoire or collection of skills and view human development as an expansion of an individual's number and range of skills. These psychologists argue that stages in human development are associated with typical ranges of skills and therefore an individual's developmental level can be assessed by comparing his or her range of skills with the range of skills shown by normal populations of an equivalent age. This approach has been described by Gunzberg (1974) and underlies the Bayley Scale of Infant Development (Bayley, 1969).

Psychologists, using a Piagetian model, see behaviour as an interaction between an individual and his or her environment and see development as an increase in the sophistication of this interaction. These psychologists argue that stages in human development are characterised by different patterns of interaction between an individual and his or her environment and that an individual's level of development can be assessed by comparing his or her interactions with the types of interactions which would be expected at different stages of human development. This approach has been discussed by Piaget (1937, 1952 and 1971) and underlies the various assessment procedures developed by Uzgaris and Hunt (1975).

Psychologists, using a radical behaviourist model, see behaviour as an adaptation to a particular environment. Human development is seen as an expansion in the range and complexities of environments within which an individual must function and an expansion of the skills to deal with these different environments. These psychologists argue that as human behaviour is adaptive and context specific, there can be no simple assessment of development. They argue that the comparison of an individual's repertoire of skills or pattern of interactions with a population norm may be seriously misleading, as it does not consider the context within which the individual exists or the purpose of the behaviour. For example "head-banging" as a form of behaviour would be difficult to classify or interpret within a skill-oriented or a Piagetian model. In a radical behaviourist model not only can head-banging be interpreted as a method by which a child can obtain attention when other methods of obtaining attention are denied, as in an institutional environment, but the psychologist can also suggest ways in which this behaviour can be modified. Thus radical behaviourists argue that behaviour is context specific and can only be understood, explained, assessed and modified in relationship to its context. Radical behaviourists do not offer a simple overall model of behaviour and therefore cannot provide a simple overall method of assessment. Rather they draw attention to the complexity of the relationships between individuals and their environments and to the need for careful and detailed descriptions of the ways in which individuals adapt to and exploit their environments and the ways this adaptation can be enhanced. Kiernan and Jones have discussed this approach and it underlies their Behavioural Assessment Battery (Kiernan and Jones, 1977, 1980(a), 1980(b) and Kiernan, 1985).

Although there is considerable debate amongst psychologists about the correct model of behaviour and the best methods for assessing behaviour, it appears that each approach has its advantages and disadvantages. Sebba (1978) argues that profoundly and multiply handicapped children should be assessed using a variety of approaches and he emphasises the need to investigate as many areas of functioning as possible. For the purposes of the present evaluation I used a pluralist approach and I used three psychological tests:

* the *Bayley Scale of Infant Development* to assess the children's repertoire of mental and psycho-motor skills.
* the *Object Scheme Scale* from the Uzgaris and Hunt assessment procedures to assess the ways in which the children interacted with objects in their environment.
* the *Behavioural Assessment Battery* devised by Kiernan

and Jones to assess the children's adaptation of their environment.

Assessment Procedures

The children admitted to the Project were assessed prior to their entry and then at six-monthly intervals during the first three years of the Project. The assessments were designed to examine whether the children were suitable for admission to the Project and to assess the impact of the Project on the children.

The Bayley Scale of Infant Development is an administratively oriented assessment battery which is commonly used to provide a global developmental age (mental and motor). The test was developed in 1969 (Bayley, 1969). It is standardised on normal children aged between 2 and 30 months. There are 163 test items on the mental scale and 81 test items on the psycho-motor scale, a total of 244 items in all. In its standardised administration only children between 2 and 30 months would be tested. However, because the test provided monthly norms in the different areas of functioning it can be adapted to assess the ways in which the skills of mentally handicapped children develop. The chronological age of the mentally handicapped child is disregarded and the child's mental and psycho-motor age is assessed by comparing his or her range of skills with those of neurologically intact children.

Like many administratively oriented assessments, the Scale does not reflect small differences in the skills of profoundly mentally handicapped children in its standard format. It is not sensitive enough to reflect these differences. However, the information collected from the tests can be broken down into individual areas of functioning. This information can then be used to analyse the strengths and weaknesses of even the most profoundly handicapped child (Foxon, 1975). There are a number of possible ways to organise items on the scale (Whitely and Krenn, 1986) but for the purpose of the present study I used the system proposed by Foxon (1975). This splits the scale into fifteen major areas of functioning, ten on the mental scale and five on the psycho-motor scale. On the mental scale the test assesses

* Auditory Skills
* Visual Skills
* Manipulation of Objects
* Visually-directed Reaching

* Visual-manual Behaviour
* Vocalisations and Productive Language
* Social Responding
* Object Constancy
* Receptive Language
* Gestural Imitation

On the psycho-motor scale the test assesses

* Head Control
* Prone Behaviour, Walking and Crawling
* Supine Behaviour
* Sitting
* Fine Motor Control

Although there are 163 items on the mental scale and 81 items on the psycho-motor scale, they are not evenly distributed across each month. For example, for the first year of life there are 107 items on the mental scale and only 56 items for the following 18 months. Similarly, the psycho-motor scale is biased in favour of the first year in that 47 items account for this period, leaving only 34 items distributed across the remaining 18 months. The scale therefore is more sensitive as an assessment instrument during the first year of life than might be expected.

The test items are presented to the children and if they make the correct response, as defined by the scale manual, it is scored as a "pass". For example, a red ring is moved across the child's visual field from left to right and the correct response for a "pass" at age 0.5 months is for the child to track the object with his or her eyes. If the child makes an incorrect response to the test or fails to respond, this is counted as a failure. The psychologist can repeat the test, if reports from parents and/or care staff indicate that the child should be able to perform this test item. However, if the child does not respond to a second presentation this is scored as a "fail" and no account is taken of the carers' statements. This can lead to inaccuracy, particularly in the case of mentally handicapped children who show skills at certain times or for certain people but not at other times or for everybody.

Although the items are arranged in ascending order of developmental difficulty, the variable performance of profoundly mentally handicapped children on this type of test means that their performance will show considerable inconsistency. It is therefore important for the psychologist to continue testing until the child has failed items covering a range of at least six months.

In the first six months the scale is a skill-oriented assessment because the items measure sensory integration and there are no verbal components. However, as the test progresses beyond this six-month period there is a strong physical and verbal component and the children have to make specific gross and fine motor movements to pass individual items. As a result the test will underestimate the level of performance of children who suffer from physical handicaps.

Although the scale has been criticised (Sebba, 1978), it remains a useful administratively oriented assessment that provides a guide to the developmental level of profoundly mentally handicapped children. As it underestimates the developmental level of the physically handicapped child, results for such children must be interpreted with caution.

The Object Schemes Scale is a functional assessment which examines specific areas of performance. It does not provide a global score of child development. Rather, it indicates the extent to which children manifest behaviour of different degrees of complexity and different developmental levels.

This scale is one of six scales developed by Uzgaris and Hunt (1975). These scales are based on a Piagetian model of cognitive development and on the assumption that as children develop they display increasingly complex interactions with their environment. Therefore, the ways in which a child uses the objects in his or her environment can be used as an indicator of the child's level of development. The scale organises these interactions in a hierarchy of increasing complexity and therefore developmental levels. For example, if a child places an object in his or her mouth this is the first and most rudimentary behaviour and is equivalent to the developmental age of two months. If the child inspects the object, then this is equivalent to the next level of development, three months and so on (see Table 10.1). Each of these schemes is defined precisely by Uzgaris and Hunt (1975) and can therefore be used as an assessment of the behaviour of either very young or profoundly mentally handicapped children.

The child is assessed in any environment in which ten objects are present. The psychologist presents one object at a time to the child and observes the interaction the child has with the object. The child is given three minutes to interact with each object. The psychologist records the various behaviours. A particular type of behaviour is scored and is said to be established if the psychologist records the child's interacting with at least three of the objects in this way. For example, if the child places three of the 10 objects in his or her mouth then the tester records this behavioural scheme as "established". To provide accurate results this test is performed with each child twice.

Table 10.1
Classification of Interactive Behaviour
in the Objects Scheme Scale

	Approximate age in months
Mouthing Objects	2
Inspecting Objects	3
Hitting Objects	4
Shaking Objects	5
Examining Objects	6
Showing Complex Behaviour towards Objects	7
Dropping or Throwing Objects	8/9
Showing Social Awareness of Objects	10
Showing Objects to Others	14
Naming Objects	18

This scale provides a functional assessment of the child's abilities and is based on the Piagetian model of cognitive development. The scale indicates the general level of development of the children and the specific type of behaviour that they manifest. Physical handicap may influence test performance. A physically handicapped child may not have the necessary motor control to interact with objects at even the most rudimentary level.

The Behavioural Assessment Battery is a functional assessment of children based on a behavioural checklist. It is the only assessment procedure that has been standardised on severely and profoundly mentally handicapped children. It was first developed in 1977 by Kiernan and Jones and they revised it in 1980. The revised version will be described here and was used in the evaluation of the children.

The battery draws on two sources of information, interviews

with care staff and/or parents and psychological assessments of the children. The tester uses the interviews and the assessments to collect information about 13 areas of development. The two sources of information are cross-checked to provide a comprehensive picture of a child's level of functioning. The battery has a very low threshold so that children who are extremely handicapped can be assessed accurately. It is particularly sensitive to small changes in levels of performance and can be used as a functional assessment because it indicates specific skills that can and should be developed. The results of the assessment are not presented as a global score but as a series of scores in each of the behavioural categories tested. From the results of these areas the child's strengths and weaknesses and level of performance can be assessed. For carers, who know the children, the detailed presentation of data provides a useful guide for the development of goal plans, etc. However, for others who want a general assessment, the level of detail means that it is difficult to present a simple summary of the results.

The areas of behavioural function sampled are

* Inspection Skills
* Tracking Skills
* Visuo-Motor Skills
* Auditory Skills
* Postural Control
* Exploratory Play
* Constructive Play
* Individual Search Strategies
* Perceptual Problem Solving
* Social Interaction
* Receptive Language Skills
* Sounds Made and Imitation of Others
* Expressive Language Abilities
* Self-Help Skills

The interviews are based on a standardised questionnaire that the tester uses to ask carers whether they have seen the child perform certain activities. The psychologist assesses the children by presenting them with a series of test items. The responses of the children to the test items are then classified in the various behavioural categories. For example, if an object is passed through the child's area of vision then the psychologist records whether the child tracks the object with his or her eyes and whether the child tracks the object with both eyes and head. The battery is a comprehensive functional assessment specifically designed for profoundly mentally handicapped children. It does not provide a global score such as mental age but rather provides an indication of the type of skills a child shows.

10.2 SEAN, BARBARA AND DAVID

In the following section I shall discuss Sean, Barbara and David. I have selected these children because they illustrate the ways in which different children responded to the Project. Sean was initially extremely difficult to test as he was very idiosyncratic in his response to test items. In the first 18 months he showed little development as measured by the three tests used. However, in the next year he started to show increased psychological development in a number of areas. Barbara was not the least able child within the Project but she made limited progress in the Project. David, on the other hand, showed immediate and large improvements after his admission into the Project and continued to do so. I present some of the data in bar chart form (Figures 10.1-10.6). The unshaded bar represents the child's performance when first tested. The black bar is the change between the first and most recent test. In the case of Sean this covers a period of two and a half years and in the cases of Barbara and David three and a half years.

Sean

Sean was a small child with obvious signs of profound and multiple handicaps. His severe physical disabilities limited his interactions with his environment.

Bayley Scale: Mental Age When Sean was first admitted he showed quite a wide range of performance on the mental age part of the Bayley Scale. However, his performance did not exceed that of a two month old child and his overall mental age was below two months when first assessed. His progress on this part of the scale was limited. He showed some consolidation in the first three months but no progress above this level. His overall mental age showed some improvement and was three months.

Psycho-motor Age Sean's performance on the psycho-motor part of the scale was initially not as good as his performance on the mental scale. He passed nearly 50% of the items in the first month but did not pass any items above that level when he was first assessed. He was performing under the two month level. When he was reassessed he had made considerable progress. He passed items in up to the 7th month and had a psycho-motor age of four months.

Behavioural Categories (Figure 10.1) When he was first assessed Sean's performance (unshaded bar) was limited by his physical handicap, for example, he did not have any head control whereas most of the other children had well-developed head control. He scored relatively well on the auditory responsiveness and object constancy and in addition passed items on manipulation of objects, visually directed reaching, social responsiveness, prone behaviour and supine behaviour. His progress (shaded bar) on the Bayley Scale was initially disappointing. He only made limited progress in auditory responsiveness and he started to show some fine motor control. However, his fifth assessment showed considerable development, particularly in the areas of visual, social and physical abilities

Objects Scheme Scale When first assessed, Sean did not interact with any of the objects he was presented with. In his fifth assessment he started to inspect and hit some objects.

Behaviour Assessment Battery (Figure 10.2) When he was first assessed Sean performed rather better on the Behaviour Assessment Battery than he did on the Bayley Scale. This may partly be accounted by the staff report element in this test. He performed well on the auditory and the expressive abilities. In his fifth test he consolidated his auditory and expressive abilities and in particular made major progress in postural control, social skills and self-help skills.

Comment When Sean was first admitted he was a profoundly mentally handicapped child performing at the bottom end of the ability range. His performance was clearly influenced by his physical handicaps. Whereas other children with similar handicaps made immediate progress following their admission to the Project, Sean's progress initially was limited especially on the Bayley Scale. On the Behavioural Assessment Battery there weresome clear areas of gain particularly in Sean's responsiveness to his environment. It was clear that Sean made progress since his admission to the Project but this progress was not as marked as that made by some of the other children.

The Psychological Development of the Children

Figure 10.1
Sean's Performance on the Bayley Scale

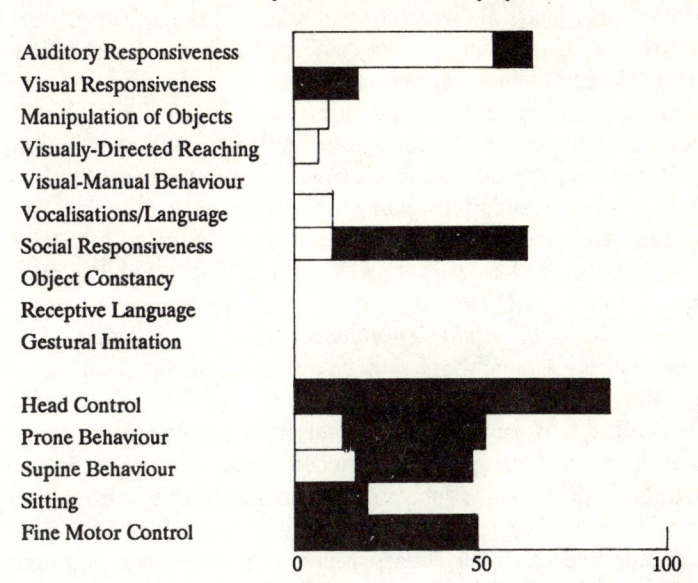

- Auditory Responsiveness
- Visual Responsiveness
- Manipulation of Objects
- Visually-Directed Reaching
- Visual-Manual Behaviour
- Vocalisations/Language
- Social Responsiveness
- Object Constancy
- Receptive Language
- Gestural Imitation

- Head Control
- Prone Behaviour
- Supine Behaviour
- Sitting
- Fine Motor Control

Percentage of Items Passed in each Behavioural Category

Figure 10.2
Sean's Behaviour on the Behavioural Assessment Battery

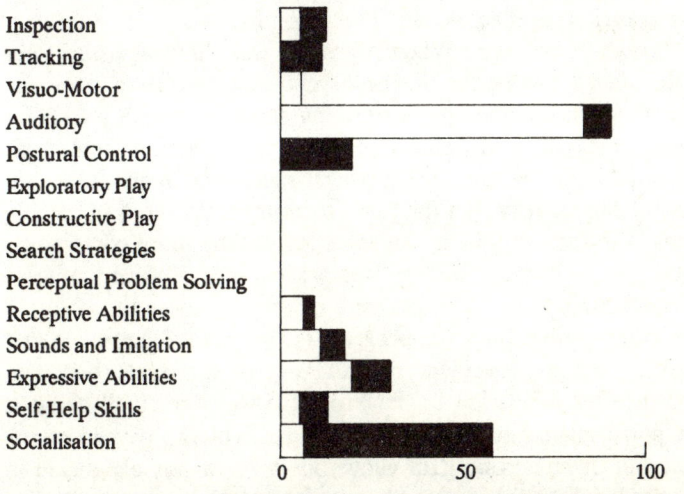

- Inspection
- Tracking
- Visuo-Motor
- Auditory
- Postural Control
- Exploratory Play
- Constructive Play
- Search Strategies
- Perceptual Problem Solving
- Receptive Abilities
- Sounds and Imitation
- Expressive Abilities
- Self-Help Skills
- Socialisation

Percentage of Items Passed in each Behavioural Category

The Psychological Development of the Children

Barbara

Barbara was 9 years old when she was admitted to the Project and had lived in hospital for five years. When I first saw Barbara she was an extremely handicapped child with clear signs of physical disability. She was severely epileptic and received anti-epileptic medication. She had no method of communication to express her needs, was only able to take fluids from a cup if it was held to her mouth and she tended to clamp her teeth on it. She had no apparent auditory dysfunction but has clear visual difficulties. Overall, Barbara was a profoundly and multiply handicapped child.

Bayley Scale of Infant Development: Mental Age When first tested Barbara's mental age was below two months. She passed over 40% of the items in the first, third and fourth month, although her performance, like that of many profoundly mentally handicapped children, was rather inconsistent. She passed items up to the sixth month but she only passed 10% of the items in the second month. She was assessed at performing at about a two and a half month level. In her 7th assessment she made some progress on the mental scale. This was more in terms of consolidation than expanding the range of her performance. For example, on the second month she now passed over 70% of the items and her performance on the fifth month had risen from 10% to over 50%. Overall she had made only limited progress and her mental age was again assessed at two and a half months.

Psycho-motor Age When Barbara was first assessed, her performance was better on the psycho-motor scale than on the mental age scale. She was performing at a four month level. Her higher level of performance on the psycho-motor scale was indicated both by the slightly wider range and more advanced level of her activity. On the psycho-motor scale she was passing items in the seventh month and was performing more consistently in the earlier months, e.g. she was passing over 50% of the items in months one to five. Her progress on the psycho-motor scale was more limited than her progress on the mental age scale and most of her improvement on this part of the scale occurred directly after admission to the Project. She made small gains in her performance in the first three months of the psycho-motor scale but there was no gain above this level or any expansion in her range of performance. She was now functioning at the five month level.

The Psychological Development of the Children

Figure 10.3
Barbara's Performance on the Bayley Scale

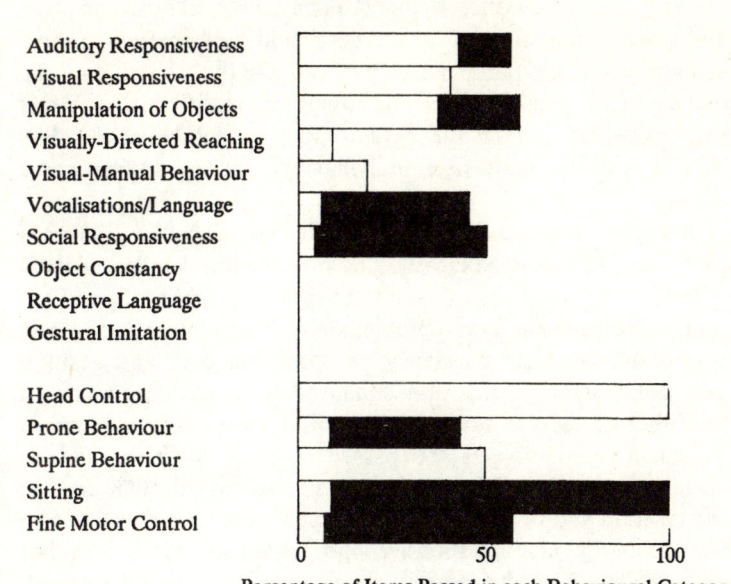

- Auditory Responsiveness
- Visual Responsiveness
- Manipulation of Objects
- Visually-Directed Reaching
- Visual-Manual Behaviour
- Vocalisations/Language
- Social Responsiveness
- Object Constancy
- Receptive Language
- Gestural Imitation

- Head Control
- Prone Behaviour
- Supine Behaviour
- Sitting
- Fine Motor Control

Percentage of Items Passed in each Behavioural Category

Figure 10.4
Barbara's Behaviour on the Behavioural Assessment Battery

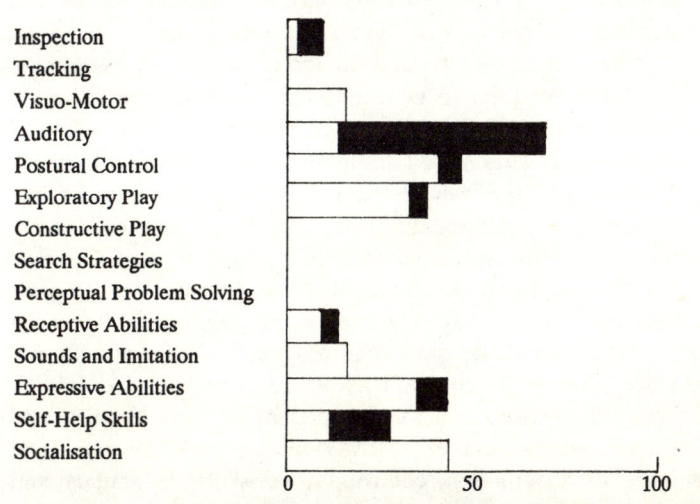

- Inspection
- Tracking
- Visuo-Motor
- Auditory
- Postural Control
- Exploratory Play
- Constructive Play
- Search Strategies
- Perceptual Problem Solving
- Receptive Abilities
- Sounds and Imitation
- Expressive Abilities
- Self-Help Skills
- Socialisation

Percentage of Items Passed in each Behavioural Category

Behavioural Categories (Figure 10.3) When Barbara was first assessed she passed items in all the behavioural categories except the more advanced ones of object constancy, receptive language and gestural imitation. However her initial performance in most categories was not particularly advanced. On the mental scale she only passed over 30% of the items in auditory and visual responsiveness and on the psycho-motor scale she passed less than 20% of the items in prone behaviour, sitting and fine motor control.

Her progress in the three and a half years since her admission to the Project could be clearly seen in the more detailed analysis of the behavioural categories of the Scale. She did not expand her range of behaviour. For example, she did not score in any new areas such as object constancy, receptive language and gestural imitation but she considerably enhanced her behaviour in most of the other areas. For example, in auditory responsiveness and in manipulation of objects she passed 60% of the items and on vocalisation and social responsiveness she passed 50% and on vocalisation and productive language she passed nearly 40%. She was generally more responsive and interacted more with her environment. On the psycho-motor scale she had developed, particularly in the area of sitting where she passed 100% of the items, and fine motor control where she passed 60% of the items in her seventh assessement.

Object Schemes Scale When Barbara was first assessed she did interact with the objects that she was presented, albeit to a limited degree. She inspected two and hit three. In her 7th assessment she had developed this form of interaction with her environment. She inspected six of the objects, hit four of them and showed more advanced behaviour by dropping or throwing four of them.

Behavioural Assessment Battery (Figure 10.4) When she was first assessed Barbara scored in most of the parts of the battery except for the more advanced areas of tracking, constructive play, search strategies and perceptual problem solving. Her progress on the battery was perhaps not as clear-cut as her progress on the Bayley Scale. She made substantial progress in auditory skills and developed her self-help skills. She also made more limited progress in postural control, inspection, exploratory play and receptive abilities and expressive abilities. But she made no progress in visuo-motor control, social skills or sounds and imitation nor had she begun to develop the more advanced skills of tracking, constructive play, search strategies and perceptual problem solving.

Comment Barbara made some progress in her three and a half years in the Project. She was more relaxed and had settled well. She had become more responsive and was more aware of her environment and was able to interact more with it. However she had shown rather less development than might have been expected considering that she was not the most dependent child within the Project. She tended to consolidate rather than expand or extend her range of skills except on the Object Schemes Scale, where she interacted with objects in a rather more advanced way.

David

When I first assessed David, he was 10 years of age and had lived in hospital for 5 years. He was an extremely handicapped child with signs of physical disability. However, he appeared very alert, particularly to auditory stimulation, although his vision seemed doubtful. He suffered from epilepsy but this was controlled by medication. He had few self-help skills. When first seen he was co-operative in feeding and recognised a cup but he had no communication skills.

Bayley Scale: Mental Age When David was first assessed on the mental part of the Bayley Scale, he was clearly a profoundly handicapped child operating in the middle range of the scale. He passed between 25% and 60% of the items up to the sixth month of development. His overall mental age was two and a half months. In his 7th assessment his progress on this scale was quite remarkable. Not only had he consolidated his performance on items in the early part of the scale, he passed all the items up to the fourth month of development, but he had also expanded his range of performance. For example, he passed all the items in the ninth month of development and he was passing over 20% of the items in the twelfth month of development. This progress was so marked that he was assessed as having a mental age of about seven and a half months, i.e. above the six month developmental level set as our "ceiling" for profound mental handicap.

Psycho-motor Age When he was first assessed David's performance on the psycho-motor part of the scale was rather better than his performance on the mental scale. He passed items in the seventh month of development and in the second month of development he passed all the items. His overall psycho-motor was four months. His progress on the psycho-motor scale was not as dramatic as his progress on the mental part of the scale. It was more a consolidation than an expansion of his range of performance. In the first four months of the scale he was now passing over 90% of the items but he did not pass any of the items above the seventh month developmental age. However, this progress was sufficient for him to be assessed as performing at the six-month level on the psycho-motor part of the scale. It was likely that his progress on this part of the scale was limited because he spent relatively long periods with his legs in plaster to help him overcome physical problems with his legs.

Behavioural Categories (Figure 10.5) When he was first assessed, David's performance on the mental part of the scale and the psycho-social part of the scale were fairly even, and typical of a profoundly mentally handicapped child performing in the middle range of the scale. For example, on the mental part of the scale he passed over 60% of the items in the auditory responsiveness and visual responsiveness but he passed less than 40% in the other categories and did not respond to the more advanced part of the scale such as object constancy, receptive language, and gestural imitation. On the psycho-motor scale he passed all the items on the head control but passed less than 40% of the items on the other parts of the scale.

In his 7th assessment his performance on the mental scale improved dramatically. He passed over 70% of the items on the scale apart from the more advanced levels such as object constancy, receptive language and gestural imitation. In these areas he began to develop behaviour. For example, in receptive language he passed nearly 60% of the items. In object constancy he passed over 40% of the items. On the psycho-motor scale he had made important advances in sitting, supine behaviour and fine motor control. He passed all the items in the sitting behavioural category, over 60% in supine behaviour and 40% in fine motor control. However, he had made no progress in pronebehaviour, walking, crawling, which indicated how his physical handicap and medical treatment had limited his progress.

Objects Scheme Scale When David was first assessed, he interacted with all the objects that he was given. He placed all ten in his mouth and inspected all ten. In addition he hit six objects, shook two, examined three and dropped or threw six. When he was assessed three and a half years later he had made significant progress both in consolidating his interaction with objects and also with extending and showing more advanced forms of

The Psychological Development of the Children

Figure 10.5
David's Performance on the Bayley Scale

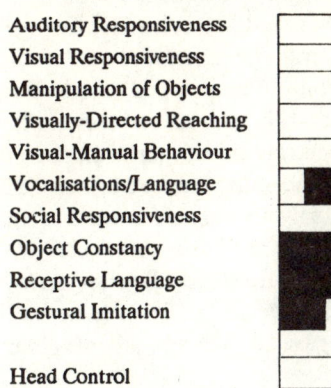

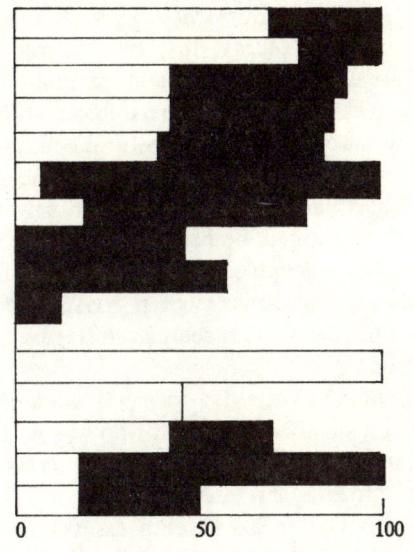

Auditory Responsiveness
Visual Responsiveness
Manipulation of Objects
Visually-Directed Reaching
Visual-Manual Behaviour
Vocalisations/Language
Social Responsiveness
Object Constancy
Receptive Language
Gestural Imitation

Head Control
Prone Behaviour
Supine Behaviour
Sitting
Fine Motor Control

Percentage of Items Passed in each Behavioural Category

Figure 10.6
David's Behaviour on the Behavioural Assessment Battery

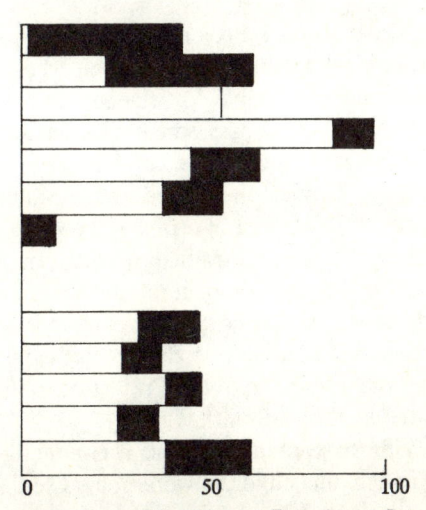

Inspection
Tracking
Visuo-Motor
Auditory
Postural Control
Exploratory Play
Constructive Play
Search Strategies
Perceptual Problem Solving
Receptive Abilities
Sounds and Imitation
Expressive Abilities
Self-Help Skills
Socialisation

Percentage of Items Passed in each Behavioural Category

interaction with objects. For example, he still put ten of the objects in his mouth and inspected them, but in addition he also hit all ten, he shook eight, examined seven and dropped or threw all ten objects. He had begun to use objects in a social context.

Behaviour Assessment Battery (Figure 10.6) When David was first assessed using the behavioural assessment battery he performed like a profoundly mentally handicapped child. His main areas of strength were in basic skills such as auditory skills, visual motor control and postural control and his performance in more advanced areas such as inspection, constructive play, search strategies and perceptual problem solving was more limited. In his 7th assessment he had made progress in most areas apart from visuo-motor control. He had also started to develop more advanced skills areas such as constructive play. However he had still not developed search strategies or perceptual problem solving.

Comment When David was first admitted he was a profoundly mentally handicapped child who was performing in the middle of the ability range. Although his progress had been restricted in some areas by his medical problems, he had made such rapid progress that in his seventh assessment he was severely rather than profoundly mentally handicapped.

10.4 SUMMARY AND COMMENT

The Croxteth Park Project is a community project for profoundly and multiply handicapped children who would traditionally only be considered suitable for placement in a health service facility. The psychological assessment was an administrative assessment that examined whether the children were profoundly and multiply mentally handicapped and an evaluative assessment that evaluated the Project in terms of the psychological progress of the children. What the evaluation did not attempt to do was to compare the development of the children with a similar group living in traditional hospital accommodation. Because of this the change within children in the Project cannot be causally linked to either the admission to the Project or to the learning environment created by the care staff.

With these points in mind it is nonetheless important to note that when the children were reassessed after six month in the Project they showed substantial improved performances. In this

The Psychological Development of the Children

six-month period most of the children showed improvements of between 20% and 33% in the various areas of assessment. After this initial increase in performance, the children continued to make progress but their improvements were more limited. Moreover no child regressed or deteriorated in terms of skills. Given the profound handicap of the children and poor medical prognosis this was quite remarkable and almost certainly related to the excellent quality of care given within the Project.

The pattern of the children's development appeared to be related to their previous care in the traditional ward environment of a hospital. It is generally accepted that this type of environment deprives children of normal forms of stimulation and experiences and can produce underfunctioning in severely and profoundly handicapped children. The initial gains of the children can be seen as an immediate result of the transfer to the more stimulating environment of the Project. Similar increases in activity and general performance have been recorded for less handicapped residents when they are discharged from institutional care (see Clarke and Clarke, 1976). The subsequent development of the children can be partially accounted for by the specific therapeutic programmes of the Project, in particular the goal plans developed for each of the children during their first year in the Project. The large initial gains of the children and their subsequent progress indicate that children who would traditionally not have been considered for placement outside a health service facility can be cared for in community-based facilities and that these children do make progress in these facilities.

The detailed analysis of the result of the assessments highlights the children's development in social skills. This appears to be related to the careful attention paid within the Project to developing the social relations of the children both through the development of the link workers scheme, and outside the Project by mobilising the informal sector of care. The link worker system ensures that each child has a R.S.W. responsible for co-ordinating his or her therapeutic programme and monitoring daily his or her living conditions. All link workers have developed strong bonds with their children. The system provides children with a close social relationship which many have not experienced before and probably accounts for much of their progress, especially in social skills.

It is possible that such a close relationship may break down and have detrimental effects if there is a high turnover of staff and a child's link worker leaves. There has been some limited evidence of this taking place. Those children, who have lost their link worker, have shown some signs of a reaction. However, this has not been long lasting and has not resulted in any measurable deterioration in their performance. Because of this potential risk, it is important that the Project continues to act as an intensive residential facility by taking children from institutional care, and placing them within a therapeutic environment for a limited period of time and then placing the majority of children in the stable and stimulating environment of permanent foster care in a family. It is only within foster families that the children will be able to experience in the long term the kind of stability and experiences that they have experienced in the short term in the Project.

11 THE CHILDREN'S QUALITY OF CARE

BIE NIO ONG, NICOLA ECCLES AND ANDY ALASZEWSKI

Ministers believe that long-stay hospitals are unsuitable places for children to grow up in because they do not provide a stimulating environment. Therefore it is important to assess the quality of care children receive in hospitals and the changes that result when children move to alternative care settings such as the Croxteth Park Project. As there is no agreed way of assessing quality of care, we shall in the first section of this chapter discuss the general issues associated with assessing quality. In the second section we shall discuss the children's daily life and in the third, child-staff interactions.

11.1 DEFINING AND MEASURING CARE

With rising demands for welfare services and limited resources available to fund them, both policy-makers and academics have become increasingly concerned with the performance of welfare agencies and the quality of their services. Street, Vinter and Perrow (1966) have argued that performance can be measured in three ways:

> * by assessing the facilities and resources available to provide care, i.e. measuring the input of resources
> * by assessing the type of care clients within the organisation receive, i.e. measuring the process of care
> * by assessing the ways in which the facility changes the client, i.e. measuring the outputs of the organisation.

Davies (1987) in her evaluation of three contrasting styles of residential provision in the Bristol area, developed measures of the "quality of life" to compare the performance of the three facilities. Davies's operational definition of quality of life was a composite measure that aimed to evaluate the performance of the facilities by assessing inputs of resources, the process of care and outputs. Inputs were defined in terms of resident:staff ratios and resident:bedroom ratios, process was defined in such terms of choice and involvement in decision-making, social contacts, day-to-day activity and outputs were measured using the STAR profile which measured "the social competence of people with learning difficulties" (p.24). Davies did not find significant changes in the output of the different services as measured by the STAR profile. She did find significant changes in terms of input of resources and process of care:

> As Table 4.11 indicates, the Wells Road Service had more staff per resident, and fewer residents per bedroom, than the hospital group, in addition to being a smaller unit ... the results suggest that the care provided by the Wells Road Service was better than that of Farleigh and Yatton Hall hospitals. (p.47)

That is possible but these results might merely indicate a higher input of resources. Without a more detailed specification and analysis of care, it is difficult to assess precisely what Davies is measuring.

The problems of interpreting Davies's measures of the quality of life indicates that perhaps at this stage in the development of research methodology she was being too ambitious. It is important to specify which particular aspect of care is being assessed and to concentrate attention on collecting detailed information about each aspect. Rather than trying to capture the overall performance of a facility, we felt it was more important to concentrate on one aspect at a time. In this chapter we focus on care, i.e. the nature and pattern of interactions between the children and the people involved in their care.

Cataldo and Risley (1974) have developed a detailed method of examining the process of care by focusing on the behaviour of residents in residential facilities and by examining the impact of staff activities on this behaviour. They examined three aspects of the care process.

* *activity*, i.e. the participation of residents in organised activities
* *interaction*, i.e the pattern of residents' interactions
* *stimulation*, i.e. the behaviour of residents and its relationship to the care environment (p.204).

In our research we started with Cataldo and Risley's approach and modified it to suit the particular nature of our study. As our research started after the admission of the first four children to Croxteth Park, the Division decided to fund a psychologist to undertake a study of the quality of care the children received in hospital. The psychologist used Cataldo and Risley's approach to the measurement of the quality of care. We replicated this study a year after the children were admitted to the Project and undertook a revised study a year later. We shall first discuss the psychologist's approach and then how and why we adjusted it.

The psychologist defined the children's activity patterns as their involvement in the routine of daily activities in the ward. As the children were on different wards, she concentrated on two of the eight children selected for transfer to the Project. She observed each child during a whole day and made records of the children's activities. She supplemented this with observations of the different activities at weekends.

The psychologist defined the children's interactions as their contact with staff and other children on the ward as well as their contact with people outside the ward. She obtained this data from two different sources. She observed the interaction patterns of four children over two days, a weekday and a weekend. She used a precoded observation schedule to make comprehensive records. The classification of staff:child interactions were:

* Feeding (including giving medication)
* Bathing (including all activities associated with bodily hygiene such as wiping a child's nose).
* Moving child
* Physical contact (defined as interactions in which a member of staff lifts or touches a child but does not move them, e.g. cuddling or stroking a child)
* Play (defined as interactions in which staff tried to amuse a child by providing a toy, or playing a game such as "peep-po").
* Talk to - close (interactions in which staff talked to child from less than two feet).
* Talk to - distant (interactions in which staff talked to child

from more than two feet).

A caring environment should provide children with a high level of stimulation. Cataldo and Risley argued that children's behaviour can be used as an indicator of the level of stimulation which they are receiving from their environment. Alert and active children are likely to be receiving stimulation from their environment. As the children were profoundly handicapped and might interact with the behaviour in very limited ways, it was important to obtain a detailed record of their behaviour. The psychologist used the following classification of behaviour:

* Vocalisation
* Vocalisation in response to a member of staff or other prior vocalisations.
* Crying
* Moaning (defined as a repetitive monotonous sound)
* Lip smacking and kissing
* Clapping (defined as repeated banging together of hands)
* Laughing
* Smiling
* Eye open/shut (recorded for children who appeared to have voluntary control over eye muscles)
* Eye direction (defined as behaviour in which child appears to focus on and watch specific object, record also made of apparent vacant gaze)
* Mouth movement (defined as behaviour in which child licked lips or moved mouth without making a noise)
* Head movement
* Head and chin banging (defined as repeated banging of head or chin on floor or striking of head and chin with hand)
* Rocking (defined as a mechanical movement such as leaning backwards and forwards when sitting or waving arms and legs in air)
* Fit (defined as any involuntary movement that appeared to be the result of a muscle spasm)
* Right Leg movement
* Left Leg movement
* Right Arm movement
* Left Arm movement
* Hands touching (defined as a position in which hand moves to touch an object, person or self, record also made if hands did not appear to touch anything).

Because of the time it took to observe and record each of these behaviours, it was impossible to observe all the time. The hospital authorities would not give the psychologist permission to video-record the children. Therefore the psychologist used a time sample approach. In the hospital study each child was observed for 12 minute periods and in each minute a 5 second period was randomly selected and the researcher recorded the child's behaviour during that 5 second period on a pre-coded sheet. Each child was observed at different times of the day in different locations.

When we started our research in the Croxteth Park Project we invited a psychology graduate to replicate the original hospital study. We found it relatively easy to observe and record activity patterns. We observed and recorded the activities of two of the children in one of the bungalows for a weekday and noted variations in the pattern at weekends.

We found it more difficult to replicate the study of interactions. In the hospital, the researcher was just another person in a ward environment of between 20 and 30 people. The situation in the Project was very different. The researcher was one of between four and five people. It was a small, intimate environment, more like a family house than a hospital ward. Furthermore, Project staff were concerned to protect the children's privacy. We therefore agreed that this researcher should have limited access to the Project and should concentrate on the interactions of the children. In this setting our researcher found it impossible to make a comprehensive record of the interactions in the Project. Instead we adopted a sampling approach. The researcher spent 12 minutes doing stimulation measures, then spent 3 minutes recording the general interactions in the bungalows. She noted the staff activities. In this way she built up a picture of the general routine of the Project and the staff/children interactions without unnecessarily intruding into the Project. She supplemented this data with information from the children's daily diaries compiled by the link workers.

We found it difficult to clearly classify interactions in the Project. In the hospital setting interactions appeared to be clearly structured and differentiated. It was fairly easy to differentiate between interactions that were designed to provide basic care and those in which staff were playing with the children. In the Project this clear differentiation did not take place, for example, the staff often played with the children while they bathed them. A straightforward quantification of our observations would have been both misleading and inaccurate. For instance, it would indicate that staff in the Project spent longer engaged in basic care activities than staff in the hospitals, but it would have been difficult to show that they performed these activities in a very different way and for very different purposes. To capture this difference we present our observation for the Project qualitatively.

We had most problems reproducing the stimulation measures. In the hospital, the psychologist was able to observe each child in several different locations and during the observation period the child stayed in this location. In the Project, the children did not stay in the same location. They were continually moved from place to place according to their care and therapy needs. Therefore it was difficult to observe their behaviour. Although the researcher in the Project used the same precoded sheets, she found it difficult, in five seconds, to observe all the behaviours specified, so she expanded the observation period to 20 seconds. Furthermore there seemed to be high levels of indeterminacy. It was often difficult to judge whether a behaviour had taken place or not.

We also had reservations about the theoretical basis of the stimulation measures. There are two major problems. The stimulation measures are based on the assumption that it is relatively easy to classify different movements or bodily positions and that these data can be used as indicators of the level of stimulation which a child is receiving from the care environment. It is not easy to classify behaviour. If a child has his arm against his body this may indicate that the child is touching himself or it may indicate that the child was doing nothing. The precise classification or interpretation depends on the context and the observer's interpretation of the child's intention. When a child suffers from profound mental handicap and/or severe physical handicaps, it may be very difficult to ascribe intention. Furthermore, even if behaviour can be unambiguously classified then there may still be problems of interpretation. For example, the stimulation measures indicated that in hospital there was a great difference in the extent to which the children vocalised. Some children were virtually silent, vocalising only 3% of observed time, whereas other children were quite noisy, vocalising 76% of the observed time. In the Project the quieter children made more noise, i.e. vocalising 13% of the observed time, whereas the noisier children were a lot quieter, vocalising 29%. It was difficult to interpret these results in terms of stimulation. Like

The Children's Quality of Care

many of the other data, they seemed to be inconsistent and not to indicate any particular pattern.

This inconsistency was not just internal it was also external. The data from the stimulation measures did not accord with the data from the children's psychological assessments. For example, the data indicated that one particular child, Mark, received more stimulation in the hospital than in the Project. For example, in hospital his left hand was touching something, e.g. 33% of the observed time whereas in the Project it was touching something only 6% of the observed time. However the psychologist's assessments indicated that Mark was making important progress in terms of hand movements. For example when he was tested in hospital on the Object Scheme Scale, he did not respond to any of the objects. When he was retested in the Project he still had no established pattern of response but he was clearly beginning to make recognisable hand and arm movements.

In view of the inconsistencies and interpretation problem, we decided not to use the stimulation measures as part of our quality of care measures. Instead we concentrated on the children's activity and interactions.

11.2 DAILY LIFE

In this section we shall examine and compare the daily life and routine of the children on the hospital ward and in the Project. We shall concentrate on the quality of care received by individual children rather than the quantity of care received by the children as a group. We shall illustrate the differences between the hospital and the Project by concentrating on the care received by one child - David.

Life on the Ward

David was an in-patient on a hospital ward in a mental handicap hospital. The following account is based on observations made during a number of weekdays. The description is therefore that of a "typical" day. At the time of the research there were 15 patients on the ward, 12 long-term care and three respite care.

6.30 (a.m.) David is woken by night staff and washed in bed. His nappy is changed, his teeth cleaned and he is dressed.

6.45 David is given a warm drink.

The Children's Quality of Care

7.30 David is taken downstairs, into the dayroom and put into his Britax chair (black plastic bucket seat, fitted into adjustable white painted steel frame, so the child can be secured into an upright or reclining seated position, by orange webbing straps). His hair is combed and his shoes put on. The night staff leave and two day staff arrive and are joined by two more for the rest of the day. They do not approach or greet the children (who are all in the day room by now) but busy themselves preparing cutlery and plates for breakfast.

8.00 Breakfast arrives from the central kitchen. (Typical menu, eggs or weetabix mashed up with milk or porridge mixed with bacon and tomatoes and liquidised. Drugs are mixed in with the breakfast.)

8.15 David is fed his breakfast. He sits in his Britax chair.

8.20 David's hands and face are washed. He remains in his chair until next activity.

8.40 David is taken out of his chair, his coat is put on and he is strapped into a wheelchair, to wait in a line facing the door, for the school bus.

9.15 The bus arrives to take the children to school (which is in the hospital grounds). Some of the children, including David had been waiting for over 20 minutes facing the door. (The children leave the ward for school at any time between 9.00 am and 9.30 am.)

9.35 The domestics arrive to clean the ward and the nurses busy themselves with sorting the laundry.

11.45 David returns from school and is taken to his Britax chair and strapped in ready to wait for his midday meal. (Typical menu, liquidised chicken, potatoes and peas followed by an orange drink and again his drugs are mixed in.)

12.05 (p.m.) David is fed his lunch.

12.30 All the children have been fed. A student nurse on placement on the ward spends about 10 minutes playing with David, squeezing a musical teddy, talking and tickling him.

12.40 Student nurse places David in his wheelchair and puts his coat on ready for school.

1.10 The school transport arrives.

3.40 David arrives back from school. He is immediately taken to the changing room where he is given a bath, a hair wash and has his nappy changed. David remains in his day clothes and is returned to the dayroom where the television is switched on.

3.55 All the children have returned from school and had been changed. The children sit or lie in front of the television. The staff have a period of relative quiet, until the evening meal arrives.

4.55 The evening meal arrives from the central kitchen and includes a bowl of soup, macaroni cheese, ice cream and jelly, ovaltine drink, together with any necessary medication.

5.00 David is fed his supper.

5.10 Following the evening meal, David and the other children are placed in front of the television and are joined by the staff, who watch it with them.

5.45 David's teeth are cleaned. He stays in front of the television. One member of staff leaves, leaving two nurses until 7.00 pm.

7.00 David still in front of television. One night staff arrives and the day nurses depart.

7.15 David still in front of television. A second member of the night staff arrives.

7.30 David given a warm milk drink.

7.40 David is taken to the changing room, has his nappy changed and is put into pyjamas. He is taken upstairs and put in bed.

8.00 All the children are in bed and the lights switched out.

9.00 David is given another drink with his night-time medication.

Further Nappy Changes The childrens' nappies are changed as a routine at *12.00 p.m.* during the night and when needed at other times.

Weekend Routine The same routine is followed except the children do not go to school.

On one of the Saturdays observed by the researcher David and five other children were taken to a children's party held at the local police station. The rest of the children remained on the ward with the television on.

On one of the Sunday afternoons, a video film was brought in by one of the staff and the children watched this and were given chocolate, sweets and fizzy drinks during the interval. On two other consecutive Sundays, the children were taken to the Lake District and to the Chester Zoo.

Comment This hospital routine was very similar to the institutional routine described by other researchers. The children were managed as a group. They were fed, washed and clothed but received little additional attention (See Alaszewski, 1986).

Life at Croxteth Park

When we conducted our follow-up study, David was living in a bungalow on Croxteth Park Estate. He shared this bungalow with one other child, Barbara. The following account is based on observations of one weekday in the bungalow.

7.00 (a.m.) Researcher arrives at bungalow. Two R.S.W.s are sitting at the dining table having a cup of tea. One is David's link worker who is reading David's diary and checking his medication sheet. David and Barbara are asleep.

7.10 David's link worker goes to the bedrooms. David and Barbara are asleep.

7.20 David's link worker goes to the bedrooms. David and Barbara are asleep.

7.30 David's link worker goes to the bedrooms. David and Barbara are asleep. He returns to the kitchen, washes up the cups and puts the washing in the washing machine, clears up the kitchen, then goes to the bathroom to prepare it for David.

7.40 David's link worker wakes David up. They have a cuddle while David is sitting up in bed and the link worker talks to David about the day. Barbara is also awake and lies in bed. The link worker has a quick talk to her as he puts away the night intercoms. An assistant link worker arrives and says hello to the children before going next door.

8.00 David's link worker checks Barbara, talks to her and then gets David and puts him in the bath. (Lots of noise and laughter can be heard coming from the bathroom.)

8.10 Link worker dresses David and takes him to his bedroom and sits him on the bed. He then checks Barbara. He gets David's wheelchair, puts him in it and takes him to the dining table. David waits at the table while his link worker prepares their breakfast. David's link worker talks to him through the open door.

8.20 The link worker goes to Barbara's bedroom to check that she is all right and then returns to sit with David. They start to eat breakfast. They talk between bites.

8.30 The R.S.W. from next door comes in for a brief chat and while he is there David grabs his link worker's bowl. (There is a lot of laughter.)

8.40 Breakfast is finished. An Assistant Link Worker puts the washing machine on. David sits in the living room listening to the radio. The link worker gets his school bag ready.

8.43 The taxi driver arrives. He goes next door to see if they

The Children's Quality of Care

are ready. The link worker fills in David's Home/School diary and David watches him.

8.50 The link worker carries David to the taxi. He goes to school with the children from the house next door. The link worker returns to see Barbara.

3.00 (p.m.) (Researcher starts afternoon observation.) Barbara sits in the side garden with David's link worker listening to the radio. She has a hat and sunglasses on.

3.15 The link worker carries Barbara into the living room. He puts her on the couch, freshens her up and puts vaseline on her face. He talks to her while he does this. (Barbara does not seem to react when her face is touched. When she first came to live in the Project, she flinched when her face was touched.) The link worker lays Barbara on a wedge and does postural drainage to clear her chest. He continues talking to her while he is doing the physiotherapy and she smiles.

3.20 The cook/domestic arrives, briefly goes into the kitchen and then goes next door.

3.23 The link worker brings the portable radio cassette into the living room. He switches on a tape of classical music. (This is Barbara's favourite music.) He continues with the postural drainage and still talks to her saying things like "you're a lovely girl" or "please take your fingers out of your mouth" when she starts chewing her fingers.

3.27 David and the two children from next door return from school in the taxi. David's link worker gets his chair out, puts him in it and gives him a drink.

3.32 Domestic/cook returns from next door, discusses what they are going to have for dinner with the link worker and starts working. Secretary comes in from office, has a quick chat and leaves the house. The link worker takes David to his room to be changed.

3.39 The link worker brings David back into living room, freshens up David and Barbara and puts David's slippers on. He then has a quick drink while David sits in his chair listening to a tape on his cassette.

3.43 The link worker lifts Barbara onto the sofa and gives her a drink. He changes the tape and asks the children which one they want. Children then listen to music.

3.55 Assistant link worker comes in to ask the link worker a question and talks briefly to the children. The link worker then takes David to the toilet. Domestic/cook goes next door.

4.00 Domestic/cook returns and carries on working in the kitchen.

4.05 The link worker starts work with David on his goal plan. (David has to focus his eyes on a biscuit, reach and take the biscuit.) Barbara stays on the couch.

4.10 The assistant link worker comes in to say goodbye and kisses the children.

4.12 The link worker records David's performance on the goal plan. He then cleans David's face. (They had been using chocolate biscuits.) The link worker switches on the television. David watches the television and the link worker takes Barbara to the bathroom.

4.27 Barbara, David and his link worker watch the television.

4.30 The link worker places David on the physio mat so that he can watch the television lying down.

4.33 The link worker lies on the mat and pulls David so that he leans on him and is more comfortable.

4.45 David and Barbara watch the television. The link worker goes through to the office.

4.47 The link worker returns and goes into kitchen. He talks to the domestic/cook while he prepares the children's medication.

4.53 The link worker returns to the living room and gives David and Barbara their fluoride drops. He places David in his wheelchair and pushes him to the dinner table. Barbara stays on the couch watching television.

5.01 The link worker and David sit at the table and start their dinner. Barbara watches the television. The link worker gets up twice to check Barbara.

5.30 David finishes his dinner. The link worker cleans David and places him in front of the television. He then gets Barbara ready for her diner and clears away physio mat.

5.38 Link worker takes David to the toilet, he brings him back to the living room and lays him on a mat in front of the television.

5.47 The link worker takes Barbara to the bathroom and changes her. He then places her in her moulded chair at the dinner table.

5.55 Barbara starts her dinner. The link worker helps her and talks to her. He gets up three times to see that David is all right.

6.26 Barbara finishes her dinner. The link worker cleans her and puts her on the settee. He sits down to mark the medication sheets.

6.30 The link worker lifts David back into his wheelchair and

The Children's Quality of Care

takes him into the kitchen. He washes up and talks to David.

6.53 The link worker brings David back into the living room. He sits next to Barbara and strokes her. He switches the television off and puts a tape in the radio/cassette. He briefly does some physiotherapy with David.

7.00 Link worker puts David on the couch next to Barbara and combs Barbara's hair.

7.02 Link worker goes next door to borrow some biscuits.

7.05 Link worker returns and sits David on his lap. They play a "rough and tumble" game.

7.10 Link worker does physiotherapy exercises with David.

7.15 Link worker takes David to the toilet.

7.20 Link worker sits David on the couch. David tries to wriggle off. Link worker fetches dry washing from the kitchen and folds it.

7.23 Link worker takes Barbara to the bathroom.

7.28 Link worker brings Barbara back and puts her on the wedge. Link worker starts postural drainage.

7.32 Link worker checks that David is all right on the settee and continues with postural drainage.

7.38 Link worker places Barbara on the settee and puts a music tape in the radio/cassette.

7.39 Link worker puts David on the mat and starts his physiotherapy exercises. He talks to him while he is carrying out the exercises.

7.54 Link worker finishes David's physiotherapy exercises and props him up with pillows so that he can relax.

7.56 David and Barbara are both asleep. The link worker makes himself a cup of tea and starts to fill in the notes.

8.40 The link worker wakes Barbara up for some more physiotherapy. David wakes up and watches.

8.45 Link worker puts David on the settee and gives him a cup of tea.

8.50 The link worker prepares the bathroom.

8.52 The link worker takes David to the bathroom.

8.58 The link worker puts David to bed. He gives him a goodnight kiss and cuddle.

9.00 The link worker fetches Barbara and gets her ready for bed.

9.05 The link worker puts Barbara to bed. He gives her a goodnight kiss and cuddle.

Weekends In the Project, the rhythm of life changed markedly during weekends and holidays. At weekends, the children "slept in" i.e. staff did not wake the children up. When they woke up, the children had a leisurely breakfast. There was also more interaction between the bungalows. Barbara usually went to her parents' house for the weekend so David spent quite a lot of time next door. Staff took the opportunity to work with each other's children and to cook and eat meals together. Weekends were not only periods of greater sociability they were also periods of leisure activities such as outings. During our second observation period, David and Barbara were taken out several times to play on inflatables which had been erected in a local park.

Comment

In the ward of the mental handicap hospital, David and the other children experienced an institutional routine. This routine has been extensively described by researchers and is characterised by a high degree of routinisation in which patients are treated as a group and staff place great emphasis on the provision of basic care, e.g. feeding, cleaning, disposing of bodily waste. As Oswin (1978) points out other needs, such as children's need for mothering and play, tend to be neglected. The structure of the routine tends to be inflexible because it is created by the staffing needs of the institution, e.g. shift-times, rather than the individual needs of the children.

In the Croxteth Park Project the rhythm of daily life was very different. There was a routine of daily activities, e.g. the taxi driver did come to collect the children for school in the morning and therefore on a school day they had to be ready, but there was also flexibility in the routine. In hospital the children were woken at the same time every day, in David's case at 6.30. In the Project, the staff, as far as possible, let the children wake up. In the morning they regularly checked whether the children were awake and only woke them when they had to, i.e. they had to have enough time to get them ready before the taxi driver arrived. The staff in the Project used the principle of normalisation as a guide to the development of the routine. The needs of the children came before those of the staff and the routine was as similar as possible to that of children of the same age living at home. In hospital the routine was a product of negotiations and relations between different groups of staff, e.g. night nurses and day nurses, ward staff and catering staff. In the Project the routine was explicitly designed. In the training, the care staff discussed the children's hospital routine and the ways in which they wanted to change it when they took responsibility for the children. Their discussions focused on the pattern of daily life in the family. The care staff accepted that most families had a routine and that was the product of both activities in the household, e.g. mealtimes, and of the relationship between the household and its environment, e.g. going to work and school. As the internal activities and external relations of the household changed so did its internal routine. The care staff tried to reproduce this flexible, changing routine within the Project.

11.3 CHILD-STAFF INTERACTIONS

In this section we shall examine staff-child interactions. As we cannot present all our data, we shall focus on interactions during the performance of basic care activities, such as bathing, and eating. We shall discuss the different style of performing these activities. In the ward environment, this style can be captured quantitatively. In the Project, the greater interpenetration of activities means that a quantitative analysis would be misleading and we present our data qualitatively.

On the Ward

The psychologist found there were high standards of physical care. The amount of time spent on these tasks varied from 51 minutes to 98 minutes per day per child. The variations related to the amount of physical care needed, the difficulty of performing this activity for a child and the availability of staff. As Table 11.1 shows the average length of time taken to perform routine activities varied between children. Ivan took the longest to feed but was the quickest to bath. Margaret took the longest to bath and change but was the quickest eater. By far the greatest proportion of staff-child interactions were related to the performance of routine care tasks (see Table 11.2 and 11.3). When staff were not involved in carrying out care routines with the children, they had other responsibilities such as sorting out laundry.

The Children's Quality of Care

Table 11.1
Average Length of Time Taken by Staff to Perform Routine Care Tasks for Each Child (Minutes)

	Eating	Bath	Wash/Change Nappy
David	12	13	7
Barbara	15	16	9
Margaret	12	20	11
Ivan	20	12	6

Table 11.2
Staff-Child Interactions on a Weekday (Minutes)

	Basic Care	Physical Contact	Play	Vocalisation Close	Vocalisation Distant
David	51.3	0	3.0	0	0.3
Barbara	74.3	1.0	0	0	0.3
Margaret	81.0	10.0	2.0	1.0	14.0
Ivan	89.3	72.0	9.0	0	0.3

Table 11.3
Staff-Child Interactions on a Weekend Day (Minutes)

	Basic Care	Physical Contact	Play	Vocalisation Close	Vocalisation Distant
David	57.0	32.0	0	0	0
Barbara	At home with parents				
Margaret	77.0	3.0	0	3.0	41.0
Ivan	95.5	75.3	0	0	0

Even at weekends, when there was less pressure of work, the staff did not devote much more time to interacting with the children. As Table 11.4 shows in the hospital basic care dominated the interactions between the children and the care staff.

Table 11.4
Basic Care Interactions as a Percentage of Total Interactions

	Weekday	Weekend
Barbara	98%	84%
David	94%	64%
Margaret	75%	62%
Ivan	52%	57%

In the Project

In the Project, basic care still played a major role. Indeed in some cases staff took longer to perform some activities such as bathing and feeding the children. However a quantified approach would be seriously misleading as it would fail to show the qualitative change in the ways in which basic care activities were performed. To do this we shall present an account of two episodes of basic care in the Project, Linda's bath/bedtime and David's meal.

Linda's bath/bedtime routine

Minute 1 Link worker carries Linda into the bathroom and starts undressing her, asking her "Are you excited?" (in singing voice) and "Bathtime for Linda."

Minute 2 Link worker puts Linda in bath and says "Throw!" and "Ready?"

Minute 3 Linda is playing with the bubbles and toys. Shared noises. Linda has her back washed.

Minute 4 Linda is lying down and link worker asks "Is it nice that?" Shared noises like "Mmmm", and when cleaning Linda's eye (she has an artificial eye) they are both laughing.

Minute 5 Linda turns on her tummy. Shared noises, like "Wow".

Minute 6 Linda on her back, having her hair washed. Link worker says "Splash!" "Where's Linda?" Linda plays with a squeeky toy and is very vocal. Link worker gets a towel while Linda splashes around.

Minute 7 Link worker holds Linda while she is swimming and both make noises.

Minute 8 Linda splashes around while the water drains away. Link worker warns her "Time to finish" and Linda gurgles.

Minute 9 Linda stands up in the bath and swings from the link worker's hands. She is shouting and both are laughing. Linda is lifted out of bath and they have a quick rough and tumble before Linda cuddles up to the link worker who asks her "Are you enjoying yourself?"

Minute 10 Linda becomes calmer and has a cuddle with her link worker. They rub noses and kiss. Link worker asks "Are you hot?" and "Are you tired?"

Minute 11 Link worker dries Linda who remains cuddled up on her lap. They talk quietly. Link worker asks "Are you ready, Linda?" and starts massaging Linda's back with warm massage oil. They do not speak and Linda is very quiet now.

Minute 12 and 13 Continuation of this quiet massage.

Minute 14 Link worker puts cream on Linda's bottom. Link worker says: "Is it cold, Linda?" and "I'm sorry", while Linda remains quiet.

Minute 15 Link worker puts a nappy on Linda who is very relaxed. Link worker talks about the day. Linda sits up and link worker praises her. They laugh. Starts drying Linda's hair.

Minute 16 Link worker wants to put Linda's nightie on but Linda protests. Link worker asks "Are you not in the mood?" and tries to coax Linda. Praises her when she puts the nightie on.

Minute 17 Link worker brushes Linda's hair, who tries to move away. Link worker praises her "She's so pretty now".

Minute 18 Link worker start to brush Linda's teeth. Link worker says "You know what's next" but Linda just plays with the brush and both laugh.

Minute 19 Linda does not want to open her mouth. Link worker coaxes her and brushes Linda's teeth. Then they both laugh.

Minute 20 Linda bites on the brush. Both laugh and finish the process.

Minute 21 Link worker carries Linda to the living room to say goodnight to Mark and his respite foster mother who kisses Linda.

Minute 22 Linda is carried to the bedroom and sits in bed alone.

Minute 23 Link worker returns with glass of water and Linda has a few little sips. Link worker asks "Don't you want a drink?", and they play peek-a-boo.

Minute 24 Linda is tucked in and has a cuddle and a kiss from her link worker. They talk quietly. Link worker leaves the room but the door remains ajar.

David's Dinnertime

Minute 1 David sits at the dinner table banging with his hand on the table while his link worker goes into the kitchen to fetch their food. He comes in to say to David "There's no milk, but do you want juice?"

Minute 2 Link worker brings in the plates and juice and starts feeding David, taking bites himself in between and says "O.K. Dave, cornbeef hash!"

Minute 3 Link worker offers David his medication and says "Another tablet, Dave?" and David takes a spoon and bangs the table.

Minute 4 Link worker offers another tablet and says "Tablet number 3." He lifts David's face to check if his bib is in place.

Minute 5 Link worker checks if Barbara is O.K. (she is on the settee) while David bangs on the table. Link worker returns to the table and asks David "It's good, hey David?" He tries David with another bite "Just beans this time, Dave, really tasty."

Minute 6 Link worker asks David if he wants a drink and offers him some juice. Praises David. David looks at his link worker and bangs the table. Link worker retorts "Is that a little hint?"

Minute 7 David pretends to take a bit, but then turns away. Link worker encourages saying "Head up, just a touch." David bangs the table and pulls a saucer.

Minute 8 David continues eating. Link worker asks "All right? Not too hot?" and "Here we go."

Minute 9 David opens his mouth willingly, and link worker asks him about school. "Do you want another drink, Dave?" David bangs the table and takes a drink, looking at the link worker.

Minute 10 Cook comes in to discuss next day's dinner and when she has gone the link worker talks about it with David.

Minute 11 David bangs the table and turns to spit his food out. Link worker comments "Maybe it was just a bit hot." He tries David's food and says "It's not too bad now."

Minute 12 David has another bit and then puts his finger in his mouth. They talk about his taxi driver.

Minute 13 David spits the next bit out. Link worker decides that he has had enough but tries to coax him by saying "Ice cream and sponge for after."

Minute 14 David has another bit, but blows the food out. Link worker says "Hey, watch my glasses" and David takes another spoonful, but then blows it out again. Link worker says "Don't

The Children's Quality of Care

spit, that's naughty."

Minute 15 Link worker wipes his glasses in the kitchen. He returns to the table and offers David another spoonful, who spits it out. Link worker tells him off "David, that's bad manners."

Minute 16 David has the last bit, and link worker asks him if he had finished and "Did you enjoy that?" David bangs the table and accepts a drink of juice.

Minute 17 Link worker goes to the kitchen to rinse David's glass while David bangs the table and looks into the kitchen.

Minute 18 Link worker brings in the puddings. "It's ice cream and sponge cake." David has a try and turns away. Link worker comments "It's very cold David, let yourself get used to it. O.K.?"

Minute 19 David puts his finger in his mouth. Link worker says "You'll soon get used to it." David is still unsure and the link worker takes a bit of his own and says "It's quite nice, David."

Minute 20 and 21 David has a bit and spits it out. Link worker says "You did that to Fred and he wasn't pleased." David has a few bites.

Minute 22 David spits out the next bit, bangs the table and turns his head backwards. Link worker asks "Not a favourite, Dave?"

Minute 23 Link worker lifts David's head to see if he is "storing" a piece of cake and then says "Let's only do the ice cream."

Minute 24 Link worker asks "Do you want a nice drink?" and David drinks some juice and coughs. His link worker reassures him. David has another sip and gets praise.

Minute 25 David has a few more sips, but coughs afterwards.

Minute 26 Cook comes in and praises David by saying "You ate all your cornbeef hash." Link worker announces to David that he is going to the bathroom to get a flannel to clean his face.

Minute 27 Link worker cleans David's face and David grumbles. Cook pops in to say goodbye.

Minute 28 Link worker clears the table and returns to brush David's hair.

Comment Staff in the hospital and the Project were caring for the same children and therefore had to perform similar activities. However they approached these tasks in very different ways. In the hospital, ward staff concentrated on basic care activities and saw these activities as an end in themselves. They tended to service the children. In the Project, care staff saw basic care as part of an overall strategy for developing the children's skills and enhancing the quality of their life. They saw basic care as an opportunity for both therapeutic and leisure activity. They often spent longer on these activities but they also performed them in a very different way. The Project staff did not treat the children as objects to be serviced, they always treated them as people to be respected. They always gave them "the benefit of the doubt". For example they talked to the children a lot, even when the children found it difficult to respond.

11.4 CONCLUSION

Many aspects of hospital organisation make hospitals unsuitable for the long-term care of children. Hospital staff may provide high-quality physical care, but as the research in hospital indicated, the provision of this care can easily become an end itself and the lives of patients dominated by a rigid routine of basic care activities. Children may spend long periods doing nothing and their emotional and social development is neglected. They may receive little affection or stimulation. When the Curtis Committee were undertaking their review in the 1940s of the public care of children, they visited a number of institutions caring for children with a mental handicap. The Committee noted the tendency, even in institutions caring for mainly non-handicapped children, for the staff to provide a reasonable standard of physical care but to show "a lack of interest in the child as an individual" (Curtis Committee, 1946). Morris (1969) found that in hospitals the needs of the person with a mental handicap were subordinated to the needs of the ward routine. Oswin (1978) quoted a nurse who commented

> if the children weren't here it would be O.K., but we don't do our work when they're around.

Similarly, King, Raynes and Tizard reported:

> In hospital, the needs of young children for affection, for individual treatment, for a variety of experiences and for continuity of relationships received little attention. Their treatment was not harsh or cruel but the environment was bleak and the atmosphere institutional. (1971, pp.192-3).

The Children's Quality of Care

Our study confirmed the findings that are beginning to emerge from other research. Small community-based residential projects can provide individualised and flexible care. For example Leonard in her review of 30 centrally funded schemes to move children with a mental handicap out of long-stay hospitals found that in most projects

> The everyday routines generally in operation in the homes reflect both flexibility and attentiveness to individual needs. Although young people, like all children, have to get up on week-day mornings in time for school or training centre, whatever their physical difficulties (provided they are not ill), week-ends give them the freedom to get up at will, in a way that was never possible in hospital. Likewise, bedtimes are adjusted to individual needs and wishes, as they would be in most "normal" homes. (Leonard, 1988, p.36)

Perhaps the major difference between care in the hospital and care in Croxteth Park Project was that in hospital the child had to fit in with a standardised package of physical care whereas in the Project the care was adjusted to suit the individual child and was designed to develop his or her physical, social and intellectual skills.

12 THE ECONOMIC COSTS

ALAN SHIELL AND KEN WRIGHT

No evaluation of new developments in community care can ever be complete without an assessment of the economic costs. Resources are always scarce in relation to unlimited human wants and choices have to be made about their best possible use. In deciding to employ resources in one activity we effectively deny ourselves the opportunity of enjoying the benefits offered by alternative uses. The value of the forgone benefits is a measure of the economic or opportunity cost of the chosen option.

If society is to make the most efficient use of its scarce resources a thorough assessment is also required of the benefits of alternative policy options. This makes it possible to identify the project which maximises the gain in benefits in relation to its cost. The costs and benefits of different options can be brought together by the technique of economic appraisal which provides a systematic framework in which they can be measured and compared (Drummond, 1980). In cost-benefit analysis (CBA) each is valued in commensurate terms, usually money, so that one may be directly offset against the other. However, the obvious difficulties of valuing the intangible benefits of social care limits the applicability of this approach.

The problem of valuing the benefits of social care programmes can be avoided if either the effects or the costs of alternative policy options are expected to be identical. Cost-effectiveness analysis (CEA) can then be used to identify the least cost/most effective option. Unfortunately alternative social care programmes will rarely have the same effects and different policies may yield, in differing amounts, a variety of benefits measured along a number of different dimensions. In this case a variant of cost-effectiveness analysis, sometimes called the

The Economic Costs

"balance-sheet" approach can be used. This method values in monetary terms the resource costs of each option and quantifies, but leaves unvalued, the benefits. It has the advantage of making both the costs and benefits of each programme explicit but leaves the difficult job of trading one off against the other to the decision-maker. Obviously a programme is efficient if it is both more effective and less costly than its alternatives. However, an option may still be considered efficient even if it is more expensive, provided that it is also more effective and the additional benefits it offers are adjudged to be worth the extra costs.

The effectiveness of the Project, in terms of the quality of care and its impact on the psychological development of the children is discussed elsewhere in this volume. In this chapter we report our estimate of the economic costs of the unit.

12.1 ASSESSING ECONOMIC COSTS

The economic approach to costing a new development such as the Project focuses on the physical resources or inputs which are required to provide the service. Once these have been identified they can be costed in a manner which reflects the benefits of using the resources in their next most valued activity. This contrasts with the approach of the accountant which tends to concentrate on the financial transactions or expenditures of his or her employing authority.

In general the workings of labour and commodity markets will tend to ensure that the price paid for a resource reflects its economic cost. To this extent the cost accounts of the unit provide a useful initial source of data. However, there are some common exceptions to the rule relating price to resource cost which prevent the accounts from showing an accurate picture of economic cost. In some cases a price may be paid for a resource which has no alternative use and therefore no economic cost. In others the prevailing price may include elements of taxation or subsidy. These often represent methods of redistributing income from one group of society to another and are not in themselves payment for resource use.

Additional inputs into the service provided by the Project will also be provided by other agencies or individuals. Health and personal social services, education and the contribution made by the children and their relatives all need to be considered to ensure that all costs are included.

The Decision Context of the Unit

The importance of the decision context stems from the definition of cost as the value of forgone alternatives. If the resource usage of a new initiative such as the Project is to be estimated it is necessary to know what net extra resources are employed in the construction, development and operation of the unit so that these can be valued according to their opportunity cost. This means identifying all resources used by the children being cared for in the unit and all the resources saved in other sectors because the new unit replaced care which would have been given elsewhere. To identify final net resource use thus requires a full specification of the alternative methods of support which would have been given if the Project had not been established.

As each of the eight children living in the unit were previously in long-stay hospital care it would be simplest to assume that this is the most likely alternative. In this case the scope to make savings is heavily dependent on the scale of Project provision. The bulk of hospital resources such as heating, lighting, medical, supervisory nursing and remedial staff are shared by a number of patients. The provision of one new Project, which would allow eight children to be discharged from hospital, is unlikely to allow many savings in these shared resources (Normand and Taylor, 1987).

The number of children resident in mental handicap hospitals has fallen rapidly over the past few years and it is public policy to develop alternative facilities, the consequence of which will be the eventual closure of these institutions. The National Development Group have also advised that no child should be admitted to a hospital for mentally handicapped people unless there are clear medical indications (National Development Group, 1977). A more likely alternative to care in the Project therefore might be a place in a small NHS or local authority community unit. These generally have less than 25 beds and tend to be situated nearer the community they serve. The problem of releasing shared resources will still arise but will not be so significant. With smaller, discrete units the expansion of Project facilities does not have to be so great before substantial savings can be made in alternative methods of care.

The Economic Costs

A simplified costing exercise might therefore compare the costs of care in the Project against the costs of a place in an equivalent community unit. Ideally, the study design would allow a comparison of the cost of care in different residential settings of children who were matched in a number of personal characteristics. Unfortunately, this was not possible because the intensity of work required to evaluate other aspects of the Project necessitated a case-study approach. Instead, information on the economic costs of a 23-place NHS unit has been taken from a report on the costs of alternative forms of NHS care written by Wright and Haycox (1985). In the opinion of one of the report's authors (KW) this unit appeared to cater for children with similar degrees of disability to those in the Project (see Table 12.1). Obviously, this method cannot control for all the extraneous factors which might explain differences in the costs of residential care and therefore, the results reported here can only be interpreted as indicative of relative costs.

Table 12.1
The Characteristics of the Two Units and Their Residents

	Croxteth Park	NHS Unit
Average number of children	8	15.6
Average age (years)	8.25	13.0
Number of children who are		
non-ambulent	7	10
physically handicapped	7	12
doubly incontinent	8	16
non-communicative	6	15
visually handicapped	5	5
aggressive	0	10
NDG class (all children)	IV	IV

Rather than focus on the average cost of the Project, there would be advantages in identifying the resource use of each resident. This would make the estimates of costs sensitive to changes in the mix of residents over time. For two reasons this proposal was rejected. For practical purposes the allocation of resource use to individuals is extremely difficult because the time of some staff members will be shared simultaneously by several children. To measure the amount of staff time devoted to each child would require close observation of the working day. This "work study" approach is time-consuming, disconcerting for the staff and may be regarded as an unwelcome intrusion into a house which is trying to provide a normal home-like environment. There are also theoretical grounds for rejecting the individual costing approach. Short-term changes in the needs of the children are, by their nature, regarded as temporary and are not matched by changes in staffing. In the long term the Project has been established to cater for a certain group of children and by and large this group will have similar characteristics despite changes in the resident population over time. Therefore, it is unlikely that individual resource use within the Project has any meaning or methodological justification.

A further consideration is the question of occupancy. It may take up to eight weeks to prepare a child for transfer from hospital into a vacancy in the Project, during which time the unit is underoccupied. However, few, if any, resources are saved, because staff work intensively with the child in hospital introducing him/her to the unit which still needs to be kept operational for the one remaining resident. Attributing the total costs of the unit only to the children resident within it would increase the average cost of care per child. This may be considered inappropriate because, once selected for transfer, the child in hospital is considered part of the unit even though he or she does not reside there. Full occupancy has been assumed because during the period under review, from April 1984 to November 1985, there was never a time when a child was not either living in the unit or living in hospital but being prepared to move to the unit.

A final concern is the time horizon over which costs should be evaluated. The simple comparative costing exercise effectively assumes that continuing care within the Project is a long-term alternative to a place in the larger NHS unit. This assumption is unrealistic because a stated objective of the Project is to prepare the children for long-term foster care. Long-term costing problems arise as soon as the unit becomes successful in this objective because the cost basis shifts from the unit itself to the costs of caring for each child over time.

The following comparative time trend of costs per child might be hypothesised (see Figure 12.1). In this case the higher costs of

The Economic Costs

care in the Project over the period *to-tf*, (where *tf* represents the time of successful placement in a foster home) are offset by the lower costs of foster care incurred in period *tf - tn*.

If the individual values of *tf* and *tn* were known then the total costs of care for each child could be calculated. However, the length of time a child needs to spend in the unit in preparation for fostering (*tf*) and the likelihood that a successful placement will be found will, in many cases, depend on factors that are beyond the control of the unit's staff. These conditions would not determine whether or not a place in the unit was offered to a child and no child would be returned to institutional care if a foster home could not be found. The focus of interest is not whether it is more costly to care for one child rather than another in the unit so much as whether over a number of years it is less costly to care for children in one way or another. The long-term costing question now becomes: for a given group of children, how do the costs of an initial stay in the Project plus any long-term foster care compare to the costs of alternative community residential facilities.

Figure 12.1
Hypothetical Comparative Time-Trend of Costs

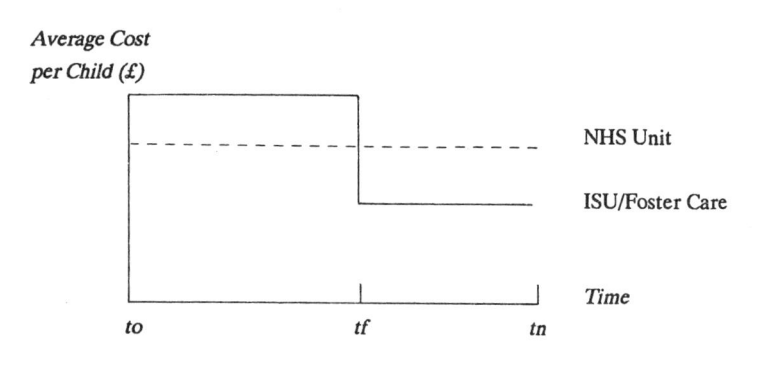

Key to time of placement in ISU
     tf time of placement in foster care
     tn period of evaluation

For some children the cost profile will initially follow the trend hypothesised in Figure 12.1. Amongst this group will be an unknown number of children who are successfully placed in foster care but for whom it becomes apparent that the arrangement can only be maintained with increased levels of social support. This may increase the costs of foster care above the level implied in Figure 12.1, perhaps significantly if occasional (or indeed permanent) readmission to residential care is eventually required. For other children the prospect of foster care is improbable and the Project is likely to become their permanent place of residence.

Therefore the period of time over which the comparative costs should be assessed becomes crucial. Setting tn too short will bias the results of the costing exercise one way or the other, either by excluding the savings made possible by foster care, or subsequently, by overestimating their magnitude. Ideally, tn should be set sufficiently high to capture each of the long-run effects.

The Project has been in operation for three years, during which time six children have been placed in foster homes. This may not be sufficient time for all the costs of foster care to become apparent and therefore the costs reported here might best be regarded as a medium-term assessment of the impact fostering has on the costs of Project-based care, to be revised in the future as experience of the operation of the unit is gained.

Identifying the Resources used by the Unit

The main real resources used in the development and operation of the Project and subsequent foster care can be categorised as follows:

* hospital - buildings and adaptations,
  - fixtures and fittings.
* Development costs
  - staff training and recruitment.
* Revenue resources
  - current running costs.
* Personal and family expenditure.
* Use of other facilities:
  - hospital in-patient stays,
  - hospital out-patient visits,
  - primary care,
  - education,
  - social services,
  - voluntary support.

* Long-term foster care:
  - preparation for a placement in foster home,
  - supervision,
  - effects on family income expenditure and leisure time,
  - continuing use of health, education and personal social services.

Capital Cost The Project is housed in four bungalows purchased and adapted specifically for the purpose. The market price of the bungalows and cost of adaptations has been revalued to 1984/85 prices and has been made comparable with the recurrent revenue expenditure by converting the total capital cost into a notional economic rent. If paid annually over the life of the building the rent would be considered as just equivalent to the initial capital cost.

Staff Development Costs The model of care practised by the Project is considered so innovative and demanding that all residential staff were required to undergo a period of five weeks training and eight weeks working with the children in hospital prior to opening the Project. This represents a large investment in staff development at significant cost before any children may be admitted.

It is difficult to estimate the cost of the development programme precisely because much of the training is done by Barnardo's own staff on a sessional basis. The cost estimate reported in the text is based on an analysis of the training programme for the second phase of the project. It includes all costs such as catering and lecture fees which can be directly attributed to the training programme, the salaries of those staff involved full-time in the programme and a proxied cost per session for those staff whose involvement was intermittent.

The cost of this initial period of training is a one-off expense and should, in theory, be treated in the same way as capital expenditure. If the total cost of this period of training and development is amortised over the lifetime of the project the annual equivalent cost becomes insignificant. For example, if the project is assumed to last for sixty years then the annual cost is less than £1,500 representing about £0.49 per child per day.

The size of this initial investment is related more to the innovative nature of the Project rather than to its current unique state. It is unlikely to diminish until many more similar units are open. For policy purposes it is important to recognise the need to invest in staff development before a new unit can become operational.

Two further sources of training cost should be noted, although neither could be quantified in this study. Replacement staff will not undergo the development programme but will receive in-service training. If staff turnover is high then the cost of this may become significant. In addition all residential staff will participate in a continuing programme of education of training. In contrast to the initial development programme, this activity is not related to a particular type of residential care and should also be a feature of alternative residential settings. However, qualitative differences in the programme may affect the relative costs.

Annual running costs The annual cost of operating the Project has been taken from the revenue accounts for 1984/85. Staff costs make up 87% of the annual expenditure and another 7% is spent on their food and travelling expenses.

Personal and family expenditure Each child is entitled to receive Mobility Allowance which is paid directly to most of the children in the Project and paid to the parents of the others. The allowance is technically a transfer payment and not a resource cost, however, it is spent on transport for visits and outings or used to purchase other personal items. This expenditure is an important component of the cost of residential care which is difficult to estimate directly but which may be proxied by the Mobility Allowance. As payment of the allowance is not dependent on the child's place of residence the costs will cancel out when comparing different modes of care.

Some families still maintain contact with their children and contribute to their care by taking them home for weekends or by purchasing toys or clothes. For completeness these costs should also be considered but, unfortunately, data on these items are not available.

Use of other facilities As the Project is a residential unit it needs to make extensive use of the statutory services for health, education and social work support (see Table 12.2). Costing the use of these services raises interesting methodological issues but, in terms of comparing the cost of alternative residential settings, the importance of these facilities should not be overemphasised.

For policy purposes, information on cost is most pertinent where it might influence decisions about alternative methods of care. This focuses attention on differences in the level of provision and type of support service required by each alternative and the likely resource implications. Irrespective of their place of residence the children currently resident in the Project would still need special education and access to acute in-patient and out-patient medical facilities. It could be argued that the development of one new Project would place no significant extra demand on these services and would therefore incur no significant additional costs. This argument is analogous to the earlier discussion about the scope to make savings in the shared resources of alternative methods of care. For example, few if any additional resources would be used if a child was admitted to hospital from the Project for an episode of acute medical care. For comparative purposes, therefore, some of these cost categories can be ignored. For example, the Project's primary care needs are met by a local group practice of general practitioners in much the same way as a normal household. The same arrangement will also prevail in other community units. In general, the demands made on the Family Practitioner Service will tend to be unrelated to the place of residence and therefore the expected costs will be the same and will cancel each other out.

Table 12.2
Use of Medical and Education Facilities

	Number
In-patient days	169
Out-patient attendances	35
Accident and emergency attendances	4
G.P. contacts	17

	No. of Children
School A	7
School B	1

Personal Social Services are an exception to this. Traditionally, social work is provided by the local authority and the costs borne by the Social Services Department. In the Project, a social work service is provided by a part-time member of Barnardo's own staff, assisted at times by the Project leader. The same social worker is also responsible for organising the foster care programme for children in the unit. The total cost, equivalent to the part-time salary plus employer's on-costs, has been apportioned between the fostering service and social work support on the basis of an estimate of the amount of time spent in each activity.

The Project also tries to make use of volunteers both to increase variety in the children's relationships and to facilitate integration with the community. Obviously voluntary services are given free or with minimal reimbursement of expenses but a valuable resource cost may be incurred if the unit's use of a volunteer's time denies another health or social service. The size of this cost depends upon the alternatives. Time given up specifically for one purpose has no alternative use and therefore no resource cost.

There is no general agreement amongst economists about how to impute a notional or shadow cost for volunteers' time. The practical problems associated with valuing this resource make the effort difficult. For this reason we have not attempted to impute a value, it is considered enough to note the importance of voluntary support.

Long-term foster care The successful placement of children into long-term foster homes incurs two distinct types of cost. The first relates to the use of a social worker's time to identify, assess and prepare prospective foster-parents for the acceptance of a child into foster care. The second category of costs arises once a child is successfully placed in foster care. This includes the costs of supervision, the effects on family income, expenditure and leisure time, the need for respite care and the continuing use made by the child of health, education and personal social services.

The foster-parents of children currently resident in the Project will be recruited from a common fostering programme which also aims to recruit parents for other children in care. Although there is some input into this programme by the social worker responsible for the children in the Project, the number of children subsequently placed is not dependent on this and, therefore, it is not possible to attribute in any meaningful sense an appropriate share of the fostering programme to each child.

To cover the costs of supervision, foster parents are entitled each week to a professional fee of £70, an attendance allowance of £20.45 and a board and lodgings payment which ranges from £28 to £48 depending upon the age of the child. The child may also be entitled to a mobility allowance of £21.40 which, as mentioned earlier, is technically a transfer payment but which can be used to proxy the final expenditures which it may finance.

To the extent that these payments are inadequate to cover the costs of supervision some family expenditure will also be redirected to support the fostered child. Opportunities for earning income may also be restricted as a result of taking on the responsibility of foster parenthood (Baldwin, 1985). In addition to these financial costs a significant proportion of the family's leisure time may have to be given over to caring for the child's physical and other needs. The problems of valuing such "informal" care have been discussed by Wright (1987), who concludes that no single valuation method is appropriate in all circumstances and that social survey techniques are essential to elicit the relative's individual attitudes to the care they provide.

The problem of valuing these costs can be avoided if it can be assumed that taking a child into foster care generates some psycho-social benefits for the family. As the decision whether or not to apply to be a foster-parent is taken voluntarily, it seems reasonable to assume, in the short term, that the benefits compensate the family for the additional costs and lost income. In this case the net cost to the family is zero.

However, foster-parenthood represents a long-term undertaking, during which real costs may become apparent at any time. Once into the process foster-parents may find it difficult to withdraw if the costs to them became higher than originally anticipated. Thus it would be important to test the assumption of zero net costs to the family as the period of evaluation is extended beyond three years to ensure that this category of economic cost is not understated. To minimise the burden felt by foster families, each is entitled to twenty-eight days of respite care. This is provided by other foster families known to the child, at a cost of £400 per annum.

Evaluating the use made of medical and education services by each child raises the problems of identifying the marginal or additional costs discussed earlier. As a result the problem can be dealt with in much the same way. If it is assumed that the use of these services will not depend upon the place of residence then it can be ignored when comparing the costs of alternative residential settings. While this assumption seems reasonable in the case of a child's schooling it is conceivably less valid in the case of health services where it is possible that a child's need for acute medical services will change slightly as a result of his or her discharge into a foster home. Unfortunately, it has not been

The Economic Costs

possible to assess the changing needs for acute medical treatment as children move between the alternative forms of care. The possibility of long-term readmission to residential care for some children was also discussed earlier. However, after three years, this situation has not occurred and therefore the question of what it might cost has not arisen.

For the personal social services the amount of support required by a child (and his or her family) is likely to change substantially after fostering. This is currently provided by the social worker who also provides an input into the common fostering programme. The amount of support required by each of the foster families varied between children and for the same child over time and the degree of variation in the amount of social support each had required prevented an accurate assessment of the costs of this service. An upper limit to the costs of a share in the common fostering programme plus subsequent social support is provided by the relevant social worker's gross salary. Rather than try to ascribe this to each child on the basis of their use of the service the annual cost has been apportioned equally between the four children found foster homes during the second year of the Project's operation.

12.2 EVALUATING THE RESOURCES USED BY THE PROJECT

It should now be apparent that there is no easy answer to the question, "What is the cost of caring for a child in the Project?" The answer will depend upon the policy context in which the question is asked and the time horizon under consideration.

Table 12.3 presents an estimate of the short-term comparative costs of residential accommodation for children who are severely and profoundly handicapped. The revenue cost of the health service unit, supplemented by the expenditures of other agencies, has been taken from the Wright and Haycox study and revalued to 1984/85 prices using an index provided by the Finance Division, D.H.S.S. A capital cost has been estimated using the cost guidelines for residential accommodation issued by the Works Division, D.H.S.S., converted to an annual rent in the same way for the Project. This includes the cost of site preparation but excludes the cost of land.

Table 12.3
Comparative Average Costs of Continuing Care

	Project £	NHS Unit £
Running costs	57.23	49.22
Capital rent *(1)*	6.04	3.40
	63.27	52.62
Personal expenditure *(2)*	3.06	3.06
Social work	0.51	0.70
	3.57	3.76
Average daily cost of continuing care *(3)*	66.84	56.38

1984/85 prices

(1) Annual equivalent rent for NHS unit excludes the cost of land.

(2) Proxied by mobility allowance.

(3) Excluding health care and education.

Excluding the costs of health care and education for the reasons cited earlier, the cost difference between the two units is almost £10.50 per day. The difference in costs can be qualified on two grounds. Although a relatively recent development, some health and local authorities are beginning to question the suitability of 24-bed units. The Jay Committee (1979) noted that views on the optimum size of residential facilities have followed a consistent trend in favour of "smallness" and that "... many people now think of small as meaning a maximum of six children in a house". This trend has continued since the publication of the Jay Report and many authorities are developing a residential service based on ordinary houses. Information on the costs of such schemes is extremely limited. In Wales the evidence from the Nimrod project (Nimrod, 1983) suggests that the cost of staffed houses for adults ranges from £39.00 to £58.00 per day (1984/85 prices) depending on whether four or six people can be accommodated in each house. To this needs to be added the residents' contribution to the running costs of the home, of £6.50 per day plus the costs of full-time education or day-services. A four-place unit would therefore cost at least £64.50 per person per day.

The Economic Costs

Secondly, care in the Project might be expected to cost more than a community unit because of the intensity of work required to prepare a child for placement in foster care. We have stressed that a full comparison would also need to consider how the costs alter once children are successfully placed in foster homes. An estimate of the costs of foster care in the medium term is presented in Table 12.4. Since this project was completed, Barnardo's have computed their own estimate of the average costs of foster care. The result, £155 per week (equivalent to £22.15 per day) is similar to the figure presented here. However, the Barnardo's estimate also includes an allowance for educational psychology, central administration and a holiday for the child.

Excluded from this is consideration of the long-term impact on personal and family costs plus an estimate of the additional costs of any health or residential care which may be required.

Interpreting the Costs

This cost data appear to substantiate the hypothesis that care in the Project is initially more expensive than a place in a larger community unit but that these costs can be reduced in the longer term as children are placed in foster care. Excluding the costs of education and health care, as these are believed to be marginal or common to all residential settings, the Project costs approximately £66.80 per child per day. Subsequent foster care for the average child costs at least £26.30 per day, subject to the qualifications noted in the text. By comparison the health service unit costs £56.40 per child per day with the prospect of future savings unlikely.

It will be recalled from Figure 12.1 that, given the time horizon over which costs will be counted (tn), the savings resulting from the Project's success in placing children in foster care will depend principally on the time required to prepare each child for placement (tf). Generally the savings will be larger the longer the period tn and the shorter the period tf provided that the unit maintains its past success and no child placed in foster care requires readmittance to residential care.

This concept can be made more tangible by following the experiences of the first eight children to be admitted to the unit to identify the appropriate values of tf and by constraining tn to three years, the length of time that the unit has been in operation.

The Economic Costs

During this period six children were placed in foster care; two after thirteen months, two after twenty-three months, one after thirty-two months and one after thirty-three months. The two remaining children have stayed in the unit since it first opened. With this information it is easy to calculate the totality of resources expended on the care of these children over the period of three years and to compare this to the cost of a hypothetical stay for an equal number of children in the NHS unit.

Table 12.4
Average Costs of Foster Care

	per child per day (£)
Preparation, placement and continuing social support *(1)*	4.07
Supervision per child *(2)*	1.18
Personal and family costs	0
Family-based respite care	1.10
Average cost per child per day	26.35

Notes

(1) Represents a portion of the responsible social worker's time divided equally amongst the four children found foster homes during the second year of the Project's operation.

(2) The families are entitled to a fixed professional fee, attendance allowance and mobility allowance. A boarding out allowance is payable which increases according to the age of the child. The reported figure represents an average of all the allowances paid to each child.

However, before these costs can be compared an allowance has to be made for the difference in the timing of the two expenditure flows. In the health service unit costs are incurred at a uniform rate throughout the three years. In the Project, higher initial costs are offset by lower expenditures towards the end of the period. The payment of interest on loans is evidence that £1 today is not valued the same as £1 in three years' time and so costs of the same nominal magnitude which are incurred at different times cannot be considered equivalent.

The process of adjusting alternative streams of costs to allow for differences in their timing is called discounting. This involves applying a weighting factor, determined by the discount rate, to costs occurring in the future so that they may be compared as if they had all occurred at the same time.

Table 12.5 presents an estimate of the three year costs of caring for the eight children first admitted to the Project both in total and discounted using the Treasury's recommended rate of 5 per cent, with equivalent figures for the costs of a hypothetical stay in the NHS unit.

Table 12.5
Total Expenditure over Three Years

Mode of Care	Unadjusted	Discounted at 5%
Project and foster care	£488,100	£457,220
NHS Unit	£493,920	£459,150

In Section 2 it was stated that the reason for calculating the long-term economic cost of the Project and comparing this with the cost of alternative residential settings was to ascertain whether, over a number of years, it was cheaper to care for children in one way or another. The table shows that after the relatively short period of three years the Project's success in placing children in foster care is having a financial effect. The relative cost advantage of the Project over long-term institutional care will continue to increase as the time horizon is extended beyond three years provided that children in foster homes do not need to be readmitted to residential care.

Although the central theme of this chapter has been the cost of the Project, the need to consider the efficiency of the unit and not just its costs was stressed in the introduction. This requires that the relative costs of care be compared to the relative outcomes so as to ascertain whether the Project is more cost-effective.

It may be that, for some children, care in the Project will always be relatively more expensive than a permanent place in a larger unit, even allowing for subsequent foster care. However, the Project may still be the most efficient option for these children if it can also be shown to be relatively more effective in improving their welfare.

12.3 CONCLUSION

It is hard to draw any firm conclusions from the results of this single study except the usual one that further research is needed to test the assumptions that have been made. For example, is the children's use of health service facilities independent of their place of residence and if it is not, can the cost consequences be ignored as marginal? Do the costs to foster parents, particularly in terms of lost leisure time, continue to be offset by the psycho-social benefits of foster parenthood in the longer term? Finally and, most importantly, can the Project maintain its success and continue to find foster homes for its children?

Without wanting to deny the importance of these questions, it does appear that over the first three years of its operation the Project was generally no more expensive than long-term care in a larger residential unit. If this experience can be maintained beyond three years then the overall efficiency of the unit depends upon the relative effectiveness of care in the different settings. Measured simply by its success in placing children in foster homes, the Project does appear significantly more effective and therefore more efficient than alternative living arrangements.

13 LESSONS FROM THE CROXTETH PARK PROJECT

ANDY ALASZEWSKI AND SUE HAYES

The Croxteth Park Project was an experimental Project which used a new model of care. From our overall assessment, it was clear that the Project was extremely successful in taking children with a profound handicap out of hospital, providing them with an intensive therapeutic programme and placing them in foster families.

In this concluding chapter, we shall concentrate on the lessons which other planners, managers and practitioners can learn from this experiment. We shall discuss the advantages and disadvantages of the Croxteth Park model and emphasise those features that should be incorporated in routine services.

13.1 SETTING UP THE PROJECT

The Bungalows

Finding suitable accommodation for a community Project is not easy. The working group, and in particular the Barnardo's architect, visited all the developments in Liverpool before they settled on four newly constructed bungalows on Croxteth Park Estate. Buying these bungalows had important advantages which included:

* *greater choice and control* The purchase of older or rented accommodation could have involved considerable expense and difficulties with planning authorities in conversion. The brand new bungalows could be used for the Project with minimal conversion and without the need for special cumbersome planning applications.

* *the attractiveness of the bungalows* Units established in rented or old properties often are in areas that are considered undesirable because of urban decay or because of various environmental hazards. Using attractive, desirable houses in areas with few environmental problems indicates that the residents are being highly valued and is an important aspect of the philosophy of normalisation.

* *operational flexibility* If the Project had been located in four separate houses then it would have had to operate as four separate sub-units. As the Project is located in two pairs of adjacent bungalows there was flexibility in the way it operated. For example, when all the children were at home the Project could operate as four sub-units, but when some of the children went home for week-end visits the Project could effectively operate as two sub-units.

There were costs involved in purchasing houses on a new housing estate. These included:

* *the small size of the houses* Houses on new estates are relatively expensive and are rather smaller than older properties. There is limited space inside them and in particular there is a lack of storage and office space in these new houses. This means that the internal environment of each house has to be carefully managed.

* *the lack of established gardens* The establishment and maintenance of gardens can be expensive. Initially the maintenance of the garden in the Project was seen as the responsibility of the care staff. However, it is important to make special provision for this so that gardens are properly maintained and to employ a part-time gardener.

* *a relative lack of community facilities* New housing estates often have few community facilities and facilities are often at some distance.

* *access problems* The children and staff in the Project used cars to travel and for them accessibility was no problem. However, parents and volunteers often did not have the same access to private transport and for them the Project was relatively inaccessible.

The Selection and Training of the Staff

The managers in Barnardo's treated selection and training as part of the same process. This approach had the advantages that it

enabled managers:
* to recruit and training staff with *the "right" attitudes*.
* *to adjust the training programme* to the specific needs of the staff that were employed.
* to use the training programme for *team development* as well as for the development of specific care skills.

Training is expensive and requires considerable input from an agency. A training programme has multiple objectives. In the training programme for the care staff there were specific issues that needed to be addressed, these included:

* *the balance between social care skills and specific inputs on medical needs and nursing skills* It is important to remember that a training programme should not only provide staff with skills but should also develop their self-confidence as carers. They need both skills and confidence when they take over the care of the children. Some information about the children's medical and nursing needs had to be provided not only to enable staff to provide proper care but also to enable them to present themselves as suitable and competent carers.

* *the process of team building* Team building is an important aspect of a training programme but it depends on proper leadership. There is a limited supply of experienced and suitably qualified people who can work as group leaders. It is difficult through a training programme to overcome this limitation.

* *subsequent training needs* Training should be considered as a continuous process. It should not be limited to the "one-off" programme for the first group of staff recruited to open the Project. The staff will need continuous training to maintain their commitment and levels of skill. New staff recruited to a Project also need basic and specialist training.

The Selection and Admission of the Children

As the Croxteth Park Project was an experimental unit, it was important that there were strict criteria for admission so that the Project could demonstrate that profoundly handicapped children could be cared for by social workers. The use of strict criteria had advantages:

* *of uniformity* All the children selected conform to the specific criteria. Therefore, individual programmes can be prepared that are suitable for these children and a body of expertise can be developed in their care.

* *for demonstrating the success of the Project* It was possible to show that in this project Barnardo's residential social workers could care for profoundly handicapped children.

However, the use of strict criteria does create problems:

* *Other professionals had different views and perceptions* of the sort of children that should be admitted to a community unit staffed by residential social workers. It was important to take into account these views so that the Project could establish good working relations and a degree of credibility. Initially some compromises had to be made. In the case of the Croxteth Park Project all the children admitted were suitable for and would benefit from admission to a community unit. However, in one case a child was admitted who was marginal in terms of a strict definition of profound mental handicap. Taking into account the views of the medical staff, the Project decided to accept the child as he would benefit from placement in the Project.

The transfer of the children from the hospitals to the Croxteth Park Project was a difficult and potentially tense period. Traditionally transfers of responsibilities have been very abrupt processes. The senior managers in the division felt it was important that the transfer of responsibility for care was not abrupt and that therefore care staff worked with the children in the hospitals before they took over full responsibility for their care. This gradual transfer has important advantages, e.g.:

* *building staff confidence* It allowed the care staff to get to know the children before they took full responsibility for their care and for the children to get to know the staff.

* *exchange of information between carers* It allowed the care staff to learn from the experience of nurses.

* *reducing the tension of the transfer* Sensitively managed, this gradual transfer allowed existing care staff to deal with the various emotional reactions that must be associated with the transfer of the care.

It is important to recognise that this transfer period is extremely sensitive and will inevitably create problems and tensions. These difficulties can be minimised by careful management but they can never be totally excluded. In particular care has to be taken with:

* *field social work support* The provision of appropriate and skilled social work support for parents concerned with making important decisions about the future care of their children.

* *the preparation of staff* from the community for work in the hospital. They will be seen as competitors and maybe seen as a threat to the competence and status of nurses in the hospital. The staff from the community unit must have adequate support while they work in the hospital taking over the responsibility of the care of the children.

* *deciding the length of the time* during which care is transferred. This will depend on the particular context, the staff in the hospital, the staff taking over care the particular needs of the child. From the experience of the Croxteth Park Project it is likely to take over a month. It is important this period of work is properly planned. It must be planned for each child and must include day and night care and weekday and weekend care.

13.2 THE OPERATION OF THE PROJECT

The establishment of a community unit such as the Croxteth Park Project is a period of excitement in which a lot of decisions have to be made rapidly. When this period is over and the Project is set up, then it can settle down into a quieter and more stable period of development. Although some of the processes of managing a project and maintaining both internal and external relations may seem less exciting, they are crucial to the success of the Project. Managers of a project must establish ways of ensuring the children receive a high quality of care and ensure that they receive proper support services.

Child Care

The central activity of a residential project is caring for its residents. The Croxteth Park Project used a formal system of care planning and a key worker system to ensure that the children received high-quality care.

Care Planning In the Croxteth Park Project each child had a six-monthly Review and a goal plan. The six-monthly review meetings set the medium- and long-term care objectives for each child. The goal plans set short-term objectives and provided the framework for day-to-day care. The planning system clearly worked well as the children made clear developmental progress and 6 of the original 8 children were placed in families within three years. This formal system of planning provided:

* *a structure for care* Each child had an explicit set of short-

and long-term objectives and all the care staff could work towards achieving these objectives.

* *a basis for monitoring the children's progress* The long- and short-term objectives could be used as a basis of assessing each child's progress.

* *a method of co-ordinating care* The regular review meetings allowed everybody involved in a child's care to meet, share information and agree care objectives. The goal planning system provided a basis for co-ordinating the day-to-day actions of carers.

It is important that care planning does not become formalised and ritualistic. To ensure this does not happen it is important that:

* objectives are *regularly reviewed and reassessed*.

* *differences in objectives* between participants are made explicit rather than concealed. If differences are concealed then the maintenance of a good relationship between participants takes precedence over the development of effective child-centred plans.

* that plans are supported by *effective records*. It is important to document the implementation of plans so that progress can be monitored and objectives reviewed.

The Link Worker System The Croxteth Park Project combined a key worker role with that of a surrogate parent to form a link worker system. The link workers took overall responsibility for planning, monitoring and assessing the care of their children and also provided as much of their day-to-day care as possible. The link worker system had important advantages for:

* *child care* It allowed for the development of bonding and attachment between a child and a member of staff.

* *communication* It provided for consistency and continuity of care.

* *management* It meant that the responsibility for the care of a specific child is clearly located with one person.

* *child's progress* The link worker can help the transition of the child into another care setting, e.g. a family placement.

There are however costs in using a link worker system. These include:

* *inflexibility* Care staff are not interchangeable. This can create difficulties in the management of resources in a Project e.g. with staff rotas, sickness and annual leave.

* *discontinuity* Staff changes can create difficulties because

some children will experience a number of changes in their link workers whereas other children will have more stability.

* *involvement* The link worker builds an intense relationship and an emotional commitment with a child. When the child moves on to another form of care the link worker will experience a serious emotional loss and even grieve for the loss of their child. It is important that this emotional commitment is recognised and that sensitive supervision and counselling is provided to enable the link worker to understand and work through his or her emotional loss.

Managing the Project

Good management is essential for the provision of good care. At times caring can be hard, unrewarding work. A good manager can provide leadership and support and can reward staff for their high levels of commitment.

In the Croxteth Park Project this managerial leadership was provided by a professionally qualified Project leader supported by two assistants. The Project leader developed a participatory style of management. This style has important advantages which include:

* *involvement* Staff are involved in the management process.

* *commitment* Staff feel committed to decisions made this way and can gain a greater understanding of the whole agency.

There are however costs in a participatory style of management. These include

* *pressure on the Project leader* It places a great strain on the Project leader who tends to act as a buffer between the care staff and the wider agency. This is a difficult role that requires a lot of skill and patience. Care staff are involved in the care of their children and may not be aware of the concerns of the wider agency and the constraints that act upon the agency. In turn the managers in the agency may not be aware of the specific problems of working within a community unit. The project leader may have to act as a go-between to try and create mutual understanding.

* *a shortage of group leaders*. The group leader's role is central to the effective management of a community project. They provide role models for the other staff. However it is a relatively low status job within social work and there are no recognised national training schemes for this type of post. It is vital that group leaders learn to combine their management and child care

roles and provide effective leadership for their care staff and effective management support for their project leader.

There are several mechanisms that can be used to support a participatory management style. These include:

* *staff supervision* It is important that staff supervision is used to monitor the performance of staff and to educate them in a proper method of performing their role.

* *staff meetings* have an important role to play in acting as a forum for discussion and communication. It is important that the limits of staff decision-making are made clear as well as those areas in which they can take decisions.

It is difficult to manage small community units and it is important that planners and managers make adequate staffing provision for such units. In particular it is important to make allowances for:

* *the intensity of the caring relationship* Individualised child care makes heavy demands on staff and they need support and resources to maintain this style of care.

* *increased workloads* caused by unexpected crises such as sickness and staff leaving or more routine events such as holidays and staff training.

Social Work Support and Fostering

All the children were informal patients in the hospitals and their transfer to the Project did not change their legal status. They were not legally in care. The local authority social service department therefore had no statutory responsibility to provide social work support for these children and their parents and social work support by the local authority for the parents and children was extremely limited while they were in hospital and remained so. When they were transferred to the Project, Barnardo's gradually took on the responsibility for providing social work support for the children and their families. It was provided either by the project leader, a qualified social worker, or by a social worker attached to the fostering service. The advantages of providing social work support within the agency are considerable. These include:

* *parental support* Parents can be supported and can be adequately prepared for the various changes that take place in their children.

* *care planning* Field social workers can provide a link

between care in a project and care in other settings such as foster families and can provide advice about the type of issues that need to be addressed in the transition.

Although the original objective of the Project was to demonstrate that the children could be cared for in a community unit staffed by social workers, the Project was not seen as a short- or long-term care facility but as one which could meet the needs of individual children and prepare them for placement in other care settings. For some, this meant placements in substitute families.

The availability of adequate social work support in the agency and in particular of a professional fostering programme was vitally important to the success of the Project. The Project could benefit from accumulated experience of the fostering programme. However, social work support needs careful planning and the impact of field social work is restricted by:

* *cost* Skilled social work is an expensive commodity that is in short supply.

* *shortages of suitably experienced staff* There is a shortage of field social workers with experience of working with children with a mental handicap and their families.

* *problems of combining social work and managerial roles* The Project tried to overcome some of the shortages of field social work support by using the Project leader to provide field social work support. There are difficulties in combining managerial and social work roles and ideally a field social worker attached to a residential Project should provide a social work service for the Project.

Involving the Informal Sector

A major objective of the Project and its staff was the involvement of the informal sector of care in the operation and care of the children. The informal sector forms an important resource and properly managed can yield considerable benefits for the children.

* *Parents* proved the most valuable resource for the children. Their involvement in the Project was vital and they could help not only with the care of their own children but also with the care of other children in the Project.

* *Volunteers* formed an important resource. They brought skills to the Project that diversified the range of experiences

available for the children. In some cases volunteers took children home and give them experiences of family life.

* *Neighbours* were an important source of help. They provided immediate support for the staff in the Project and a pattern of reciprocity developed.

The informal sector is essentially "unreliable". Parents, volunteers and neighbours do not have the same sort of contractual relationships as employees of Barnardo's nor do they have the same legal obligation to provide services as do statutory agencies, such as the Health Service. Therefore it is important to encourage and foster the development of relationships with the informal sector. Members of the informal sector must be allowed to choose what sort of relationship they want with the Project. Some will choose to have a fairly minimal relationship, for example, some parents or neighbours will maintain a friendly but distant relationship. Other parents and neighbours will choose to develop close relationships and for them the Project will become a significant place. Therefore it is important:

* *not to expect too much of the informal sector* In particular it is important that a project does not become reliant or in any way dependent on the informal sector. Volunteers, parents, neighbours should be an optional extra and should not be seen as an alternative to members of staff.

* *not to be over-ambitious* In relation to both volunteers and neighbours, the Croxteth Park Project may have started by being rather over-ambitious, for example the volunteers started at the same time as the staff. This seemed a good idea at the time but it did not work. Volunteers should have started after the staff and only when the staff had become familiar with their own role and confident with their own activities. Similarly the Project initially tried to actively encourage the involvement of neighbours. Only a few neighbours responded to this approach. It would have been better to start with a lower profile and aim to blend as inconspicuously as possible into the neighbourhood.

* *to ensure access* Access is vital for members of the informal sector. Although neighbours by definition live locally, few parents and few volunteers will live within walking distance. Some parents and volunteers will have their own transport but, for those that do not, access is vital and a project should provide or arrange transport.

Support from Statutory Services

The support of statutory services is vital for the success of a community unit. A community unit is essentially a residential Project and should concentrate on the provision of residential care. It should not attempt to become a 24-hour care environment. If it does, it will merely become a mini-institution. Although agencies such as the local education authority and the district health authority are legally obliged to provide services such as education and health care this legal obligation does not necessarily guarantee that adequate and appropriate services are provided. It is important to develop effective communication with these agencies so that the right sort of support is provided.

* *Education departments* are legally obliged to provide education but it is necessary to ensure that educational programmes fit with the care programmes developed within a project. It is vital to develop continuous liaison with teachers in the schools so that there is a consistency of care planning.

* *General medical practitioners and dental practitioners* are obliged through their contracts with family practitioner committees to provide general medical and dental services. Neither type of practitioner normally has specialist expertise of providing services for profoundly mentally handicapped children and again it is important to liaise with them and where necessary to seek more specialist advice.

* *Specialist health care* It is important to establish good working relationships with the hospital medical and nursing staff. This can be done through establishing credibility with the hospital and as a result obtaining rapid access to hospital facilities for the care and treatment of the children.

* *Physiotherapy* is vital for the development of profoundly handicapped children. There is a shortage of community physiotherapists. Some basic physiotherapy can be provided by care staff but it is also important to ensure that physiotherapy is provided regularly and if necessary to make funds available for a physiotherapy service.

* *Speech therapy and visual and hearing assessments* are also important. Again there may be difficulties in obtaining these services and a special provision may have to be made to obtain them.

13.3 CONTEXT OF CARE

The transfer of children to a community unit such as the Croxteth Park Project raises a number of wider issues that need to be addressed. These include the long-term future of the children, the need for monitoring the progress of the children and the role of research in the operation of a Project.

Agency Support

A Project such as the Croxteth Park Project should not operate in isolation within an agency but should operate within a framework that offers support both to the Project and to the parents and children. The Croxteth Park Project was able to make use of a range of support services with the Barnardo's N.W. Division.

* *Care Planning* The Project was offered as part of a total care plan for each child which could involve the use of the resources of the fostering project.

* *Psychology* The Project could make use of the psychology expertise of the Division and this was particularly important in the development of the goal plans.

* *Training* The Project could make use of the staff development and training resources of the division.

Long-Term Care Issues

The placement of severely dependent children in community units requires consideration of their long-term care. Children with a profound mental handicap will continue to be dependent and will have very special needs as adults. It is important that any subsequent care environment is at least of equal standard to the care that they received in a community-based project. It is therefore important that the future of these children is protected as they continue into adult life and that they are placed in an environment that both enhances their development and provides them with security in the long term. Family placement is one way in which this security and support can be provided into young adulthood.

The Psychological Assessment and Follow-Up of the Children

It is important for an experimental Project to monitor the

progress of the children by undertaking regular psychological assessments. There are advantages for applying this approach to the care of the children in more routine facilities for:

* *child assessment* It enables the response of the children to a project and therefore the efficacy of a project to be routinely monitored.

* *care planning* It provides information that can be used in the development of individual programmes for the children.

There are difficulties in routinely assessing children caused by:

* *shortages of skilled staff* Psychological assessment is a highly skilled activity and there is very limited expertise in this area.

* *lack of assessment procedures* The existing psychological assessment tests are relatively crude. They need to be refined and developed to provide more sensitive instruments for the assessment of the children's progress.

Research

The Croxteth Park Project was subject to intensive research by a whole range of specialists. This research was important in the development of the Project.

* *Staff motivation* Research made the staff conscious that their activities were important and were worth the attention of researchers.

* *Information* Research provided an independent source of information about the Project and its development that could be used to monitor its overall progress and to identify areas that required management attention.

However, such intensive research does create problems.

* *Intrusion* The research can be intrusive and can increase the pressure on the staff. It is important that researchers establish close relationships with care staff and take care to explain the objectives and purposes of their work.

* *Anxiety* can develop about the results of the research. It is important that there is an early feedback of the results of the research to both care staff and the managers so that they can see the type of information that is being collected and the use to which this information is being put.

* *Feedback* Researchers may identify what they believe to be problems developing within the Project. It is important that regular meetings take place between researchers and senior managers to act as a forum for discussion of the results of the

research and how this information can be used to modify and develop practice in the Project.

13.4 FINAL COMMENT

The Croxteth Park Project has been a successful service innovation. It shows how a well thought out Project which is grounded in an explicit ideology such as normalisation, with careful planning and an adequate range of support services can enhance the development of children with a profound mental handicap.

The success of such a Project depends on the context within which it is established. It is important that managers not only believe in the philosophy and principles but demonstrate this belief. In addition they must be willing to take the necessary risks which are essential to its success.

Managers have been able to create a "cycle of success" in the Croxteth Park Project. In hospital the children were often placed in a deprived and unstimulating environment. They tended to be withdrawn and passive and were often treated as objects to be serviced. In the Project the children have experienced an exciting and challenging environment. They have been stimulated and have become socially responsive. This responsiveness has made the children attractive and interesting. The children have become the focus of attention and activity. They are socially valued.

BIBLIOGRAPHY

Abbott, M. and Chamberlain, P. (1986) "Living Together", *Nursing Times*, March 5, pp. 49-51.

Abrams, P. (1977) "Community Care: Some Research Problems and Priorities", *Policy and Politics*, 6, pp. 125-151.

Abrams, P. (1984) "Realities of neighbourhood care: The interactions between statutory, voluntary and informal social care," (ed. M. Bulmer), *Policy and Politics*, 12, pp. 413-428.

Alaszewski, A. (1978) "The Situation of Nursing Administrators in Hospitals for the Mentally Handicapped: Problems in Measuring and Evaluating the Quality of Care," *Social Science and Medicine*, 12, pp. 91-97.

Alaszewski, A. (1986) *Institutional Care and the Mentally Handicapped: The Mental Handicap Hospital*, Croom Helm.

Alaszewski, A., Ong, B.N. and Lovett, S. (1986) *Residential Care for Children who are Profoundly Mentally Handicapped*, Barnardo's.

Alaszewski, A. and Chappell, A. (1987) *The Development of Community Relations on a New-Owner Occupier Housing Estate*, Barnardo's.

Alaszewski, A. and Ong, B.N. (1987) "Community Care for Profoundly Mentally Handicapped Children", N. Malin (ed) *Reassessing Community Care*, Croom Helm.

Allen, P. (1983) "Training Direct Care Staff", A. Shearer (ed) *An Ordinary Life: Issues and Strategies for Training Staff for Community Mental Handicap Services*, King's Fund Project Paper, No. 42.

Atkinson, D. and Ward, L. (1987) "Friends and Neighbours: Relationships and opportunities in the community for people with a mental handicap", N. Malin (ed) *Reassessing*

Bibliography

Community Care, Croom Helm.
Ayer, S. (1984) "Handicapped Children in the Community", Occasional Paper, *Nursing Times*, 80, pp. 66-69.
Ayer, S. and Alaszewski, A. (1986) *Community Care and the Mentally Handicapped: Services for Mothers and their Mentally Handicapped Children*, Croom Helm.
Baldwin, S. (1985) *The Costs of Caring*, Routledge and Kegan Paul.
Bamford, T. (1982) *Managing Social Work*, Tavistock.
Barclay Committee (1982) *Social Workers: Their Role and Tasks, The Report of a Working Party set up in October 1980 at the request of the Secretary of State for Social Services by the National Institute for Social work under the Chairmanship of Mr Peter M. Barclay*, Bedford Square Press.
Barnardo's Child Care Services (1968) *A Brief Review of the Child Care and Special Education Services*, Barnardo's.
Barnardo's (1981a) *A Review of Barnardo's Child Care Work*, Barnardo's.
Barnardo's (1981b) *Report of the Working Party on the Use of Volunteers*, Barnardo's.
Barnardo's (1981c) *Intensive Support Unit for Mentally Handicapped Children*, Barnardo's.
Barnardo's N.W. Division (1986) *Management for Group Leaders in Residential Settings*, Barnardo's N.W. Division.
Barnes, J.A. (1976) *The Ethics of Inquiry in Social Science*, Oxford University Press, Oxford.
Barnes, J.A. (1979) *Who Should Know What? Social Science, Privacy and Ethics*, Penguin.
Barr, H. (1987) *Perspectives on Training for Residential Work*, Study 8, Central Council for Education and Training in Social Work.
Baumeister, A.A. (1965) "The usefulness of the IQ with severely retarded individuals: A reply to MacAndrew and Edgerton", *American Journal of Mental Deficiency*, 69, pp. 881-882.
Bayley, A. (1969) *Bayley Scale of Infant Development*, New York, Psychological Corporation.
Belknap, I. (1956) *Human Problems of a State Mental Hospital*, McGraw-Hill, New York.
Benson, J.K. (1975) "The Inter-Organisational Network as a Political Economy", *Administrative Science Quarterly*, 20, pp. 229-249.
Berger, M. and Yule, W. (1985) "IQ tests and Assessment", A.M.

Bibliography

Clarke, A.D.B. Clarke and J. Berg, (eds.) *Mental Deficiency: The Changing Outlook*, 4th ed., Methuen.

Berkson, G. and Landesman-Dwyer, S. (1977) "Behavioral Research on Severe and Profound Mental Retardation (1955-1974)", *American Journal of Mental Deficiency*, 81, pp. 428-454.

Bodenham, J. (1983) "Freedom of Choice for the Mentally Handicapped", *British Journal of Occupational Therapy*, 46, pp. 356-9.

Bolton Neighbourhood Network Scheme (1984) *A Comprehensive Response to the "Care in the Community" Initiative, Bolton*, Bolton Metropolitan Borough and Bolton Health Authority.

Booth, T.A. (1981) "Collaboration between Health and Social Services", *Policy and Politics*, 9, pp. 23-49 and pp. 205-226.

Bowlby, J. (1951) *Maternal Care and Mental Health*, World Health Organization, Geneva.

Bowlby, J. (1965) *Child Care and the Growth of Love*, Penguin.

Bowlby, J. (1979) *The Making and Breaking of Affectionate Bonds*, Tavistock.

British Association of Social Work/Residential Care Association (1976) "How can residential and field social workers co-operate?" *Social Work Today*, 7, pp. 346-348, 2nd September.

Bulmer, M. (1979) "Concepts in the Analysis of Qualitative Data", *Sociological Review*, 27, pp. 651-677.

Burlingham, D. and Freud, A. (1944a) *Young Children in War Time*, Allen and Unwin.

Burlingham, D. and Freud, A. (1944b) *Infants without Families: The Case for and Against Residential Nurseries*, Allen and Unwin.

Campaign for the Mentally Handicapped (1974) *Fostering Mentally Handicapped Children: Is it Feasible?* Enquiry Paper No. 3, CMH.

Carle, N. (1981) "Key Concepts: Individual Programme Plans", *CMH Newsletter*, 26, pp. 3-4.

Cataldo, M.F. and Risley, T.R. (1974) "Evaluation of Living Environments: The Manifest of Description of Ward Activities", Davidson P.O., F.W. Clarke, and L.A. Hamerlynck, (eds.) *Evaluation in Behavioural Programs in Community Residential and School Settings*, Champaign, Illinois, Research Press, 1974.

Cherniss, C. (1980) *Professional Burnout in Human Service Organisations*, Praeger.

Clarke, A.D.B. and Clarke, A.M. (1984) "Mental Subnormality in

Bibliography

Childhood and Adulthood", A. Gale and A.J. Chapman (eds.) *Psychology and Social Problems*, John Wiley and Sons, Chichester.

Clarke, A.M. and Clarke, A.D.B. (1976) *Early Experience: Myth and Evidence*, Open Books.

Cochrane, A.L. (1972) *Effectiveness and Efficiency: Random Reflections on Health Services*, The Nuffield Provincial Hospital Trust.

Community Care (1981) "What Social Workers Think: A Survey of Facts and Opinions, *Community Care*, pp. 10-13, 16th April.

Community Care (1983) "£9m offer to help bring children into the community", *Community Care*, p. 3, 13th January.

Community Care (1983) "Tories spend more on voluntary organisations", *Community Care*, p.3, 8th December.

Court Committee (1976) *Fit for the Future: Report of the Committee on Child Health Services*, (Chairman, Professor S.D.M. Court), Cmnd. 6684-I, HMSO.

Crick, M. (1985) "'Training' the Anthropological Self: Quizzical Reflections on Field Work, Tourism and the Ludic", *Social Analysis*, 17, pp. 71-92.

Curtis Committee (1946) *Report of the Care of Children Committee*, Cmd. 6922, HMSO.

Dartington, T., Miller, E.J. and Gwynne, G.V. (1981) *A Life Together: The Distribution of Attitudes around the Disabled*, Tavistock.

Davies, L. (1982) *Residential Care: A Community Resource*, Heinmann.

Davies, L. (1987) *Quality, Costs and "An Ordinary Life": Comparing the costs and Quality of Different Residential Services for People with Mental Handicap*, King's Fund Project Paper, Number 67.

Davis, L. (1978) "A Case for Consultancy", *Social Work Today*, 10, p. 27, 10th October.

Dexter, L.A. (1964) "On the Politics and Sociology of Stupidity in our Society", H.S. Becker (ed) *The Other Side: Perspectives on Deviance*, The Free Press, New York.

D.H.S.S. (1971) *Better Services for the Mentally Handicapped*, Cmnd. 4683, HMSO.

D.H.S.S. (1972) *Management Arrangements for the Reorganised NHS England*, Cmnd. 5055, HMSO.

D.H.S.S. (1973) *Collaboration between the NHS and Local Government: A Report from the Working Party*, HMSO.

D.H.S.S. (1976) *Priorities in Health and Personal Social Services in England*, HMSO.

D.H.S.S. (1980) *Mental Handicap: Progress, Problems and Priorities: A Review of Mental Handicap Services in England since the 1971 White Paper*, HMSO.

D.H.S.S. (1981a) *Residential Facilities for Mentally Handicapped Children, Mental Health Building Pamphlet 1*, D.H.S.S.

D.H.S.S. (1981b) *Health Service Residential Accommodation for Severely Mentally Handicapped People: How to Make the Most of Current Design Guidance, Mental Health Building Pamphlet 2*, D.H.S.S.

D.H.S.S. (1981c) *Opportunities for Volunteering: Consultation Paper*, D.H.S.S.

D.H.S.S. (1981d) *Care in the Community: A Consultative Document on Moving Resources for Care in England*, HMSO.

D.H.S.S. (1981e) *Care in Action: A Handbook of Policies and Priorities for Health and Personal Social Services in England*, D.H.S.S.

D.H.S.S. (1983) *Care in the Community and Joint Finance*, Circular HC (83) 6/LAC (83)5, D.H.S.S.

D.H.S.S. (1985) *Government Response to the Second Report from the Social Services Committee, 1984-85 Session, Community Care*, Cmnd. 9674, HMSO.

Dodson, G. and Ong, B.N. (1987) *The Link Worker System: An Innovation in Child Care Practice*, Barnardo's.

Donges, G.S. (1982) *Policy Making for the Mentally Handicapped*, Gower.

Douglas, R. and Payne, C. (1985) "When your efforts are not valued", *Social Work Today*, 17, p. 21, 21st October.

Drummond, M.F. (1980) *Principles of Economic Appraisal in Health Care*, Blackwell, Oxford.

Dunham, J. (1978) "Staff stress in residential work", *Social Work Today*, pp. 18-19, 25 July.

Elliott, D. (1980) "Some Current Issues in Residential Work: Implications for the Social Work Task", R. Walton and D. Elliott (eds.) *Residential Care: A Reading in Current Theory and Practice*, Pergamon.

ENB and CCETSW (1986) *Report of the ENB/CCETSW Joint Working Group, Cooperation in Qualifying and Post-Qualifying Training: Mental Handicap*, ENB/CCETSW.

Fahlberg, V. (1979) *Attachment and Separation: Putting the Pieces Together*, Michigan Department of Social Services, Michigan,

Bibliography

Illinois.
Faludi, A. (1973) *Planning Theory*, Pergamon.
Felce, D. (1983) "Selection, recruitment and promotion", A. Shearer, (ed) *An Ordinary Life*, King's Fund Project Paper, no. 42.
Felce, D., Mansell, J., de Kock, V., Toogood, S. and Jenkins, J. (1984) "Housing for Severely Mentally Handicapped Adults", *Hospital and Health Services Review*, pp. 170-4.
Finch, J. and Groves, D. (1980) "Community Care and the Family: A Case for Equal Opportunities", *Journal of Social Policy*, 9, pp. 487-511.
Foxon, T. (1975) "Assessment of the Profoundly Handicapped Child using Normal Infant Development Tests", J. Hogg, T. Foxon and R.E. Remington, "Research into the Assessment and Remediation of Behavioural Deficit in Profoundly Retarded Multiply Handicapped Children", Third Report to the DES, Hester Adrian Research Centre, University of Manchester, Manchester.
Freire, P. (1985) *The Politics of Education*, MacMillan.
Friend, J.K., Power, J.M. and Yewlett, C.S.L. (1974) *Public Planning: The Intercorporate Dimension*, Tavistock.
Geertz, C. (1973) *The Interpretation of Cultures*, Basic Books, New York.
Glennerster, H., Korman, N. and Marslen-Wilson, F. (1983a) *Planning for Priority Groups*, Martin Robertson.
Glennerster, H., Korman, N. and Marslen-Wilson, F. (1983b) Plans and Practice: The Participants' Views, *Public Administration*, 61, pp. 265-281.
Graham, H. (1983) "Do her Answers fit his Questions: Women and the Survey Methods", E. Gamarnikov et al. (eds.) *The Public and the Private*, Heinemann.
Griaule, M. (1965) *Conversations with Ogotomelli: An Introduction to Dogan Religious Ideas*, Oxford University Press.
Grunewald, K. (1986) "The Intellectually Handicapped in Sweden - New Legislation in a bid for Normalisation", *Current Sweden*, no. 345, pp. 1-10.
The Guardian (1985) "Move to switch care services worries charities", p. 2, 11th June.
Gunzberg, H.G. (1974) "The Education of the Mentally Handicapped Child", A.M. Clarke and A.D.B. Clarke (eds.) *Mental Deficiency: The Changing Outlook*, 3th ed., Methuen.
Hall, R. et al. (1977) "Patterns of Inter-Organisational

Relationships," *Administrative Science Quarterly*, 22, pp. 457-475.

Harbridge E. (1981) "Can community care win the resources tug-o-war?", *Community Care*, pp. 12-14, 16th July.

Harrison, L. and Tether, P. (1987) "The Co-ordination of U.K. Policy on Alcohol and Tobacco", *Policy and Politics*, 15, pp. 77-90.

Hayes, S. and Alaszewski, A., (1986) *Setting up a Community Unit: Lessons the Dr Barnardo's Intensive Support Unit in Liverpool*, Barnardo's.

Haywood, S., Redmore, E. and Ostle, B. (1979) *Case Studies in N.H.S. Management*, Institute for Health Studies, University of Hull, Hull.

Health and Social Service Journal (1985) "Community Care - No More Cash", News Section, 95, p. 1492, 20 November.

Health and Social Service Journal (1985) Community Care - No More Cash, News Section, 95, p. 1492, 20 November.

Heywood, J.S. (1978) *Children in Care: The Development of the Service for the Deprived Child*, Routledge and Kegan Paul, 3rd edition.

Hogg, J. and Mittler, P.J. (1980) "Recent Research in Mental Handicap: Issues and Perspective", J. Hogg and P. J. Mittler (eds.) *Advances in Mental Handicap Research, Vol.1*, John Wiley, Chichester.

Hunt, L. (1985) "Implementation of Policies for Community Care: The D.H.S.S. Contribution", *Health Trends*, 17, pp. 4-6.

Hutton, W.D., Talkington, L.W. and Altman, R. (1973) "Concomitants of multiple sensory deficit", *Perceptual and Motor Skills*, 37, pp. 740-742.

Jay Committee (1979) *Report of the Committee of Enquiry into Mental Handicap Nursing and Care, Vol. I* (Chairman Peggy Jay), Cmnd. 7468-I, HMSO.

Johnson, C.G. (1982) "Risks in the Publication of Fieldwork", J. E. Seiber (ed) *The Ethics of Social Research: Fieldwork Regulation and Publication*, Springer-Verlag, New York.

Joint Working Group (1981) of TRRL and Gwent County Council, The Application of *Accessibility Measures in Gwent: Travel to Hospitals and Shops*, TRRL Laboratories Report 994.

Jones, K. (1975) *Opening the Door: A Study of New Policies for the Mentally Handicapped*, Routledge and Kegan Paul.

Jones, K. and Fowles, A.J. (1984) *Ideas on Institutions: Analysing* the Literature on Long-Term Care and Custody, Routledge and Kegan Paul.

Jones M. C. (1983) *Behaviour Problems in Handicapped Children: The Beech Tree House Approach*, Souvenir Press.

Jones, S.R. (1981) *Accessibility Measures: A Literature Review*, TRRL Laboratories Report 967.

Jones, S.R. (1984) *Accessibility and Public Transport*, TRRL Supplementary Report 832.

Kendall, A. and Moss, P. (1972) *Integration or Segregation? The Future of Educational Services for Mentally Handicapped Children*, Campaign for the Mentally Handicapped.

Kiernan, C.C. (1985) "Behaviour Modification", A.M. Clarke, A.D.B. Clarke and J. Berg, (eds.) *Mental Deficiency: The Outlook*, 4th ed., Methuen.

Kiernan, C.C. and Jones, M. (1977) *Behavioural Assessment Battery*, Windsor, N.F.E.R.

Kiernan, C.C. and Jones, M. (1980a) *Behavioural Assessment Battery*, 2nd ed., N.F.E.R., Windsor

Kiernan, C.C. and Jones, M. (1980b) "Behavioural Assessment Battery", J. Hogg and P. Mittler (eds.) *Advances in Mental Handicap Research, Vol. 1*, John Wiley and Sons, Chichester.

King, R.D., Raynes, N.V. and Tizard, J. (1971) *Patterns of Residential Care: Sociological Studies in Institutions for Handicapped Children*, Routledge and Kegan Paul.

Korman, N. and Glennerster, H. (1985) *Closing a Hospital: The Darenth Park Project*, Bedford Square Press.

Landesman-Dwyer, S. (1974) "A description and modification of the behavior of nonambulatory, profoundly mentally retarded children", Unpublished doctoral thesis, University of Washington.

Leonard, A. (1988) *Out of Hospital: A Survey of 30 Centrally Funded Schemes Providing Alternative Care for Children with Mental Handicaps*, Department of Social Policy and Social Work, University of York, York.

Lipsky, M. (1980) *Street-Level Bureaucracy*, Russell Sage Foundation, New York.

Liverpool Area Health Authority (1979) *Area Strategic Plan, 1979/80-1988/89*, Liverpool A.H.A.

Lyle, J.G. (1959) "The Effect of an Instutional Environment upon the Verbal Development of Institutional Children, (1) Verbal Intelligence", *Journal of Mental Deficiency Research*, 3, pp. 122-8.

Lyle, J.G. (1960) "The Effect of an Institutional Environment upon the Verbal Development of Imbecile Children, (3), The Brooklands Residential Family Unit", *Journal of Mental Deficiency Research*, 4, pp. 14-23.

McKeganey, N. and Hunter, D. (1986) "Only Connect... Tightrope Walking and Joint Working in the Care of the Elderly", *Policy and Politics*, 14, pp. 335-360.

McKeown, R.A. (1980) "Who goes home? A study of discharges from three hospitals for the mentally handicapped", *Apex*, 8, pp. 78-9.

McKinlay, J.B. (1975) "Clients and Organizations", J.B. McKinlay (ed.), *Processing People: Cases in Organizational Behaviour*, Holt, Reinhart and Winston, New York.

MacLachlan, R. (1986) "Martin: A Success Story", *Community Care*, 11th December.

Mansell, J., Felce, D., Jenkins, J. de Kock, V. and Toogood, S. (n.d.) "Staffed House for 8 Mentally Handicapped Adults" unpublished paper, Health Care Education Research Team, Southampton University, Southampton.

Mansell, J., Felce, D., Jenkins, J., de Kock,V., and Toogood, S. (1987) *Developing Staffed Housing for People with Mental Handicaps*, Costello.

MENCAP (1985) *The MENCAP Homes Foundation. The Development of Residential Services for Mentally Handicapped People*, MENCAP.

Milgram, S. (1974) *Obedience to Authority: An Experimental View*, Harper and Row.

Miller, E.J. and Gwynne, G.V. (1971) *A Life Apart: A Pilot Study of Residential Institutions for the Physically Handicapped*, Tavistock.

Miller, E.J. and Rice, A.K. (1967) *Systems of Organisation*, Tavistock.

Mitchell, C.G.B. and Town, S.W. (1977) *Accessibility of Various Social Groups to Different Activities*, TRRL Supplementary Report 258.

Mittler, P. (1979) *People not Patients: Problems and Policies in Mental Handicap*, Methuen.

Morris, C. (1984) *The Permanency Principle in Child Care Social Work*, University of East Anglia, Norwich.

Morris, P. (1969) *Put Away: A Sociological Study of Institutions for the Mentally Retarded*, Routledge and Kegan Paul.

National Association of Health Authorities (1985) *Progress in*

Bibliography

Partnership, NAHA.
National Development Group for the Mentally Handicapped (1977) *Mentally Handicapped Children: A Plan for Action*, Pamphlet No. 2, HMSO.
Nichter, M. (1984) "Project Community Diagnosis: Participatory Research as a First Step towards Community Involvement in Primary Health Care", *Social Science and Medicine*, 19, pp. 237-252.
Nimrod (1983) *Preliminary Information on Costs*, Mental Handicap in Wales, Applied Research Unit, Cardiff.
Normand, C. and Taylor, P. (1987) *The Decline in Patient Numbers in Mental Handicap Hospitals: How the Cost Savings Should be Calculated*, Centre for Health Economics, University of York, Discussion Paper No. 26, York.
Oakley, A. (1981) "Interviewing Women: A Contradiction in Terms", H. Roberts (ed) *Doing Feminist Research*, Routledge and Kegan Paul.
O'Brien, J. and Tyne, A. (1981) *The Principle of Normalisation: A Foundation for Effective Services*, CMH.
Ong, B.N. and Alaszewski, A. (1988) "Nurses No Longer Required", *Nursing Times*, 84, pp. 41-43, 29th June.
Oswin, M. (1978) *Children Living in Long-Stay Hospitals*, Spastics International Medical Publications.
Parsloe, P. (1981) *Social Services Area Teams*, Allen and Unwin.
Parsloe, P. and Hill, M. (1978) "Supervision and Accountability", O. Stevenson and P. Parsloe, *Social Services Teams: the Practioners' View*, D.H.S.S.
Payne, C. (1977) "In Residence: Investing in Residential Skills", *Social Work Today*, 8, p. 19, 22nd March.
Payne, C. and Scott J. (1982) *Developing Supervision of Teams in Field and Residential Social Work: Part 1*, National Institute for Social Work, Paper No. 12.
Piaget, J. (1937) "Principal Factors Determining Intellectual Evolution from Childhood to Adult Life", in *Factors Determining Human Behavior*, Harvard Tercentenary Publication, No.1, Harvard University Press, Cambridge, Mass.
Piaget, J. (1952) *The Origins of Intelligence in Children*, International University Press, New York.
Piaget, J. (1971) *Science of Education and the Psychology of the Child*, Viking Press, New York.
Pickup, L. (1984) *Residential Mobility among Council Tenants: The*

Role of Transport and Accessibility, TRRL Laboratory Report 1100.

Pines, A. (1983) "On Burnout and the Buffering Effect of Social Support", B. A. Farber (ed) *Stress and the Human Services*, Pergamon.

Pritchard, C. (1983) "Bridge of Sighs", *Social Work Today*, 14, pp. 10-12.

Potter, P. (1986) *Long-Term Residential Child Care: The Positive Approach*, Social Work Monograph, University of East Anglia, Norwich.

Prosser, H. (1976) *Perspectives on Residential Child Care: An Annotated Bibliography*, NFER.

Personal Social Services Research Unit (1985) "Housing and Support Services", *Care in the Community*, P.S.S.R.U., pp. 3-7 University of Kent, Winter, Canterbury.

Personal Social Services Research Unit (1987) *Care in the Community*, P.S.S.R.U., University of Kent, Spring, Canterbury.

Race, D. (1987) "Normalisation: Theory and Practice", N. Malin (ed) *Reassessing Community Care*, Croom Helm.

Raynes, N.V. and Sumpton, R.C. (1987) "Training Needs of Community Staff: What Do They Want?" *Mental Handicap*, 15, pp. 95-97.

Raynes, N.V., Pratt, M.W. and Roses, S. (1979) *Organisational Structure and the Care of the Mentally Retarded*, Croom Helm.

Righton, P. (1985) "A Fairer Share of Learning", *Social Work Today*, 16, p. 19, 18th March.

Ross, R.T. and Boroskin, A. (1972) "Are IQ's Below 30 Meaningful?", *Mental Retardation*, 10, p. 24.

Royal Commission on the Law Relating to Mental Illness and Mental Deficiency (1957) *Report*, Cmnd. 769, HMSO.

Sebba, J. (1978) "A System for Assessment and Intervention for Pre-School Profoundly Retarded Multiply Handicapped Children", unpublished M.Ed. thesis, University of Manchester, Manchester.

Seebohm Committee *Report (1968) Report of the Committee on Local Authority and Allied Personal Social Services*, Cmnd. 3803, HMSO.

Sellitz, C. et al. (1965) *Research Methods in Social Relations*, Methuen.

Shakespeare, R. (1970) "Severely Subnormal Children", P.J. Mittler (ed) *The Psychological Assessment of Mental and*

Bibliography

Physical Handicaps, Tavistock Publications in association with Methuen.

Shearer, A. (1980) *Handicapped Children in Residential Care: A Study of Policy Failure*, Bedford Square Press.

Shearer, A. (1981) *Bringing Mentally Handicapped Children Out of Hospital*, King's Fund Project Paper, no. 30.

Shearer, A. (1983) (ed) *An Ordinary Life: Issues and Strategies for Training Staff for Community Mental Handicap Services*, King's Fund Project Paper, no. 42.

Shearer, A. (1984) *Progress in Bringing Mentally Handicapped Children Out of Hospital*, Report 84/85, King's Fund Centre.

Shearer, A. (1986) *Building Community with People with Mental Handicaps, Their Families and Friends*, Campaign for People with Mental Handicaps and the King Edward's Hospital Fund.

Shiell, A. and Wright, K. (1988) "The Economic Costs of a Normal Life: The Case of Dr Barnardo's Intensive Support Unit", *Mental Handicap Research*, 1, pp. 91-101.

Sieber, J.E. (1982) "Ethnographic Fieldwork and Beneficial Reciprocity", J.E. Sieber (ed) *The Ethics of Social Research: Fieldwork, Regulation and Publication*, Springer-Verlag, New York.

Smith, G. (1986) "Service Delivery Issues", *The Quarterly Journal of Social Affairs*, 2, pp. 265-283.

Smith, G. and Cantley, C. (1985) *Assessing Health Care: A Study in Organisational Evaluation*, Open University Press, Milton Keynes.

Social Services Committee (1985) *Second Report, Session 1984-85, Community Care with Special Reference to Adult Mentally Ill and Mentally Handicapped People*, Volume 1, Report, House of Commons, HC 13-1, HMSO.

Spencer, D.A. (1979) "The Rehabilitation of the Long-Stay Mentally Handicapped Adult in Hospital", *Teaching and Training*, 17, pp. 46-49.

Stanley, L. and Wise, S. (1983) *Breaking Out: Feminist Consciousness and Feminist Research*, Routledge and Kegan Paul.

Stark, J.A., McGee, J.J. and Menolascino, F.J. (1984) *International Handbook of Community Services for the Mentally Retarded*, Lawrence Erlbaum Associates.

Street, D., Vinter, R.D. and Perrow, C. (1966) *Organization for Treatment*, The Free Press, New York.

Tizard, J. (1964) *Community Services for the Mentally*

Handicapped, Oxford University Press, Oxford.

Tizard, J. (1975) "The Quality of Residential Care for Retarded Children", J. Tizard, I. Sinclair and R.V.G. Clarke (eds) *Varieties of Residential Experience*, Routledge and Kegan Paul.

Tizard, J. and Grad, J.C. (1961) *The Mentally Handicapped and Their Families: A Social Survey*, Oxford University Press.

Tizard, J., Sinclair, I. and Clarke, R.V.G. (1975) *Varieties of Residential Experience*, Routledge and Kegan Paul.

Towell, D. (1980) *An Ordinary Life: Comprehensive Locally-based Residential Services for Mentally Handicapped People*, King's Fund Project Paper, no. 24.

Towell, D. (1983) "Foreward", A. Shearer (ed) *An Ordinary Life*, King's Fund Project Paper, no. 42.

Towell, D. (1985) "Health and Social Services Relationships in the Reform of Long Term Care: Giving Impetus to Social Service Development", *British Journal of Social Work*, 15, pp. 451-456.

Tyne, A. (1987) "Shaping Community Services: The Impact of an Idea", N. Malin (ed) *Reassessing Community Care*, Croom Helm.

Uzgaris, I.C. and Hunt, M.McV. (1975) *Assessment in Infancy: Ordinal Scale of Psychology Development*, University of Illinois Press, Urbana, Illinois.

Wagner Committee (1988) *Residential Care: A Positive Choice: Report of the Independent Review of Residential Care*, HMSO.

Walton, R. and Elliott, D. (1980)(eds.) *Residential Care: A Reader in Current Theory and Practice*, Pergamon.

Ward, L. (1984a) *Planning for People: Developing a Local Service for People with Mental Handicap, Recruiting and Training Staff*, King's Fund Project Paper, no. 47.

Ward, L. (1984b) "Feeding back for Feelings", *Social Work Today*, 15, p. 20, 16th July.

Warnock Committee (1978) *Special Educational Needs: Report of the Committee of Enquiry into the Education of Handicapped Children and Young People*, (Chairman, Mrs H.M. Warnock), Cmnd. 7212, HMSO.

Wax, M.L. (1982) "Research Reciprocity Rather than Informed Consent in Fieldwork", J.E. Sieber (ed) *The Ethics of Social Research: Fieldwork, Regulation and Publication*, Springer-Verlag, New York.

Webb A. and Wistow G. (1982) *Whither State Welfare? Policy and Implementation in the Personal Social Services 1979-80*, Royal Institute of Public Administration.

Bibliography

Welsh Office (1983) *All Wales Strategy for the Development of Services for People who are Mentally Handicapped*, Welsh Office.

Whiteley, J.H. and Krenn, M. (1986) "Uses of the Bayley Mental Scale with Nonambulatory Profoundly Mentally Retarded Children", *American Journal of Mental Deficiency*, 90, pp. 425-431.

Whyte, W.F. (1955) *Street Corner Society*, University of Chicago Press, Chicago.

Wildavsky, A. (1979) *The Art and Craft of Policy Analysis*, Macmillan.

Williamson, D.A. (1978) "Perceptions of Staff Supervision in the Probation Service", *British Journal of Social Work*, 8.

Willmott P. (1963) *The Evolution of a Community: A Study of Dagenham after Forty Years*, Routledge and Kegan Paul.

Wistow, G. and Fuller, S. (1983) *Joint Planning in Perspective: The NAHA Survey of Collaboration, 1976-1982, National Association of Health Authorities*, Centre for Research in Social Policy, Loughborough University, Loughborough.

Wistow, G. and Fuller, S.(1986) *Collaboration Since Restructuring: The 1984 Survey of Joint Planning and Joint Finance*, Centre for Research in Social Policy, Loughborough University.

Wolfensberger, W. (1972) *The Principle of Normalisation in Human Services,* National Institute on Mental Retardation, Toronto.

Wolfensberger, W. (1974) *The Origins and Nature of Institutions*, Syracuse University, Human Policy Press, Syracuse, New York.

Wolfensberger, W. (1983) "Social Role Valorization: A Proposed New Term for the Principle of Normalisation", *Mental Retardation*, 21, 6, pp. 234-9.

Wright, G. (1978) "A model of supervision for residential staff", *Social Work Today*, 9, pp. 20-23, 25th July.

Wright, G. (1980) "The right way to staff supervision", *Social Work Today*, 11, pp. 216-27, 6th May.

Wright, K.G. (1987) *The Economics of Informal Care of the Elderly*, Centre for Health Economics, University of York, Discussion Paper no. 23, York.

Wright, K.G. and Shiell, A. (1987) *Assessing the Economic Costs of a Community Unit: The Case of Dr Barnardo's Intensive Support Unit, Centre for Health Economics*, Centre for Health Economics, University of York, Discussion Paper 31, York.

Wright, K.G. and Haycox, A.R. (1985) *Costs of Alternative Forms of NHS Care for Mentally Handicapped Persons*, Centre for Health Economics, University of York, York.

Young, M.D. and Willmott, P. (1957) *Family and Kinship in East London*, Routledge and Kegan Paul.

INDEX

Abbott, M. 77, 103, 112, 281
Abrams, P. 161, 281
Alaszewski, A. 1, 5, 12-48, 56-204, 227-248, 267-280, 281, 282, 287, 288
Allen, P. 78-79, 281
Allen, Lady 13
Atkinson, D. 163, 281
Altman, R. 207, 282, 287
Ayer, S. 1, 162, 282

Baldwin, S. 260, 282
Bamford, T. 140, 282
Barclay Committee 16-17, 118-119, 282
Barnardo's 3, 12, 16, 36, 49, 58, 59, 103-4, 121-2, 164-5, 282
Barnes, J.A. 31, 37, 38, 282
Barr, H. 16, 282
Baumeister, A.A. 207, 282
Bayley, A. 208, 210, 282
Becker, H.S. 284
Belknap, I. 139, 282
Benson, J.K. 184, 282
Berg, J 288
Berger, M. 208, 283
Berkson, G. 207, 283
Bodenham, J. 58, 283

Bolton Neighbourhood Network Scheme 77, 283
Booth, T.A. 183, 283
Boroskin, A. 207
Bowlby, J. 13, 14, 122, 283
British Association of Social Work 118, 283
Bulmer, M. 281, 283
Burlingham, D. 13, 283

Campaign for the Mentally Handicapped 24, 283
Cantley, C. 34, 35, 36, 183, 292
Carle, N. 120, 283
Cataldo, M.F. 228-30, 283
CCETSW 285
Chapman, A.J, 283
Chappell, A. 3, 5, 160-182, 281
Chamberlain, P. 77, 104, 113, 281
Cherniss, C. 133, 283
Clarke, A.D.B. 206, 225, 283, 284, 287
Clarke, A.M. 206, 225, 283, 284, 287
Clarke, F.W. 283
Clarke, R.V.G. 34, 293
Cochrane, A.L., 284

Index

Court Committee 21, 119, 284
Crick, M. 43, 45, 284
Curtis Committee 14, 15, 18, 247, 284

Dartington, T. 141, 284
Davidson, P.O. 283
Davies, L. 228, 284
Davis, L. 141, 284
Dexter, L.A. 23, 284
D.H.S.S. 3, 20, 36, 38, 40-49, 100-1, 110, 160-2, 183, 284, 287
Dodson, G. 4, 5, 7-11, 30, 48-56, 117-138, 285
Donges, G.S. 184, 285
Douglas, R. 142, 285
Drummond, M.F. 25, 285
Dunham, J. 141, 285

Eccles, N. 2, 227-248
Elliott, D. 117, 285, 293
ENB 285
ENCOR 10, 22, 23

Fahlberg, V. 122, 286
Faludi, A. 182, 286
Farber, B.A. 291
Felce, D. 100, 286, 289
Finch, J. 162, 286
Fowles, A.J. 97, 288
Foxon, T. J. 210, 286
Freire, P. 42, 286
Freud, A. 13, 14, 283
Friend, J.K. 183, 286
Fuller, S. 183, 294

Gale, A. 283
Gamarmkov, E. 286
Geertz, C. 40, 286
Glennerster, H. 57-58, 74, 283, 286, 288

Graham, H. 42, 286
Griaule, M. 44, 286
Groves, D. 162, 286
Grunewald, K. 22, 286
Gunzberg, H. 208, 287
Gwynne, G.V. 141, 284, 289

Hall, R. 184, 287
Hamerlynck, L.A. 283
Harbridge, E., 287
Harrison, L. 183, 287
Haycox, A.R. 252, 261, 295
Hayes, S. 4, 5, 267-280, 287
Haywood, S. 58, 287
Heywood, J.S. 13, 15, 287
Hill, M. 140, 290
Hogg, J. 207, 208, 287
Hunt, L. 208, 210, 212, 287
Hunt, M. McV. 208, 212, 293
Hunter, D. 183, 289
Hutton, W.D. 207, 287

Jay Committee 21, 25-27, 99, 120, 262, 287
Jenkins, J. 286, 289
Johnson, C.G. 45, 287
Jones, K. 97, 288
Jones, M. 206, 209, 214, 288
Jones M.C. 39, 288
Jones, S.R. 112, 288

Kendall, A. 4, 7-11, 24, 30, 48-56, 288
Kiernan, C.C. 206, 209, 214, 288
King, R.D. 20, 29, 34, 247, 288
King's Fund, 24, 185
Kock, de, V 286, 289
Korman, N. 57-58, 74, 286, 288
Krenn, M. 210, 294

297

Index

Landesman-Dwyer, S. 205, 207, 283, 288
Leonard, A. 248, 288
Lipsky, M. 139, 288
Liverpool Area Health Authority 106, 289
Lovett, S. 2, 5, 68, 205-226, 281
Lyle, J.G. 33, 289

McGee, J.J. 23
McKeganey, N. 184, 289
McKeown, R.A. 58, 289
McKinlay, J.B. 139, 289
MacLachlan, R. 5, 289
Malin, N. 291, 293
Mansell, J. 3, 100, 285, 289
Marslen-Wilson, F. 286
MENCAP 185-6, 289
Menolascino, F.J. 23, 293
Milgram, S. 31, 289
Miller, E.J. 141, 143, 284, 289
Mittler, P.J. 207-8, 288, 289, 292
Mitchell, C.G.B. 112, 290
MORC 10
Morris, A. 3, 183-204
Morris, C. 16, 290
Morris, P. 34, 247, 290
Moss, P. 24, 288

National Association of Health Authorities 184, 290
National Children's Homes 12
National Development Group for the Mentally Handicapped 251, 290
Nichter, M. 42, 290
Nimrod 262, 290
Normand, C. 251, 290

Oakley, A. 42, 290
O'Brien, J. 98-99, 187, 290
O'Neill, D. 14
Ong, B.N. 2, 5, 30-48, 56-159, 197, 227-248, 281, 285, 290
Ostle, B. 58, 287
Oswin, M. 240, 247, 290

Parsloe, P. 139, 140, 290
Payne, C. 141, 142, 285, 290
Perrow, C. 227, 293
Piaget, J. 208, 290
Pickup, L. 112, 291
Pines, A. 133, 291
Pratt, M.W. 34
Pritchard, C. 141, 291
Potter, P. 15, 17, 291
Power, J.M. 286
Prosser, H. 15-16, 291
Personal Social Services Research Unit 77-78, 99, 109, 110, 291

Race, D. 25, 291
Raynes, N.V. 20, 29, 34, 79, 147, 288, 291
Redmore, E. 58, 287
Residential Care Association 118, 283
Rice, A.K. 143, 289
Righton, P. 141, 291
Risley, T.R. 228-30, 283
Roses, S. 34, 291
Ross, R.T. 207, 291
Roughton, H. 12-29, 47, 139-59
Royal Commission into the Law Relating to Mental Illness and Mental Deficiency 19, 291

Scott, J. 142, 290
Sebba, J. 68, 209, 212, 291

Index

Seebohm Committee 16, 292
Sellitz, C. 32, 292
Shakespeare, R. 207, 292
Shearer, A. 19, 21, 59, 99, 162-3, 185, 281, 292, 293
Shiell, A. 2, 5, 249-266, 292, 295
Sieber, J.E. 287, 292, 294
Sinclair, I. 34, 293
Smith, G. 34, 35, 36, 183, 292
Social Services Committee 17, 109, 292
Spencer, D.A. 58, 292
Stanley, L. 43, 293
Stark, J.A. 23, 293
Stevenson, O 290
Street, D. 227, 293
Sumpton, R.C. 79, 291

Talkington, L.W. 207, 287
Tether, P. 183, 287
Tizard, J. 18, 19, 20, 29, 33, 247, 293
Toogood, S. 286, 289
Towell, D. 25, 76, 77, 186, 293
Town, S.W. 112, 290
Tyne, A. 24, 98-99, 187, 290, 293

Uzgaris, I.C. 208, 210, 212, 293

Vinter, R.D. 227, 293

Wagner, G. xvii-xviii
Wagner Committee 17-18, 28, 119, 141, 155, 293
Walton, R. 117, 285, 293
Ward, L. 3, 77-78, 141, 163, 281, 293
Warnock Committee 119, 293
Wax, M.L. 32, 294
Webb, A., 183, 294
Welsh Office 76, 119-20, 294
Whiteley, J.H. 210, 294
Whyte, W.F. 33, 294
Wildavsky, A. 182-3, 294
Williamson, D.A. 141, 294
Willmott P. 161, 294, 295
Wise, S. 43, 293
Wistow, G. 183, 294
Wolfensberger, W. 10, 22, 23, 24, 25, 294
Wright, G. 142, 294, 292, 295
Wright, K.G. 2, 5, 249-266, 295

Yewlett, C.S.L. 286
Young, M.D. 161, 295
Young, Sir George 99
Yule, W. 208, 283